Intermittent Fasting for Women 101

The Ultimate Step-by-Step Guide for Weight Loss, Even If You Are Over 50, with the Keto Diet, 16/8 Method and Self-Cleansing Through the Metabolic Process of Autophagy.

Jennifer Cook

Table of Contents

Introduction

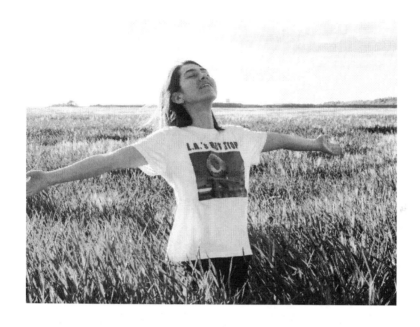

Congratulations on purchasing *Intermittent Fasting for Women 101* and thank you for doing so.

Intermittent fasting is a method of eating that any woman can use to lose weight and achieve a healthier body. Unlike in traditional fasting, intermittent fasting allows you to cycle between periods of eating and not eating. Doing so activates a biological process called autophagy that cleans out the toxins from your cells. When triggered by intermittent fasting, as well as other methods such as the keto diet and exercise, autophagy slowly gets you habituated into healthier lifestyle habits like eating nutritious foods and exercising.

This book doesn't skip a beat in telling you how to make intermittent fasting a seamless part of your life. The book even covers topics like how pregnant women and women over 50 can successfully start intermittent fasting. Read on to change how you look and feel for good.

Most people get interested in intermittent fasting and autophagy because of what they can do for their weight and for the natural detox. While these benefits are something you don't want to miss, it is astounding how intermittent fasting can do even more for you. When we talk about the many positive effects intermittent fasting has on your body, we can split them into two categories: effects that you see fairly soon and long-term effects that are even more important in the grand scheme of things.

The effects that you see early on include younger-looking skin with a glow, weight loss, and an increase in the energy you have to spend every day. These alone usually convince people that they should do intermittent fasting to trigger autophagy, but there is even more it can do for them. That's because the advanced autophagy you will see in your body will cause all the operations in your body to run much more smoothly, leading to countless positive effects like less inflammation, lower cholesterol, lowered risk of cancer, lowered risk of heart disease, and a massive reduction in the knots and tangles in the brain linked to neurodegenerative diseases like Alzheimer's disease and Parkinson's disease.

It would be hard to decide which effects to your health you care about more, but fortunately, there is no need for you to choose. If you follow a new routine of intermittent fasting, you will get all of them — and this book has everything you could possibly need to know about how to get there.

There are plenty of books on this subject on the market, thanks again for choosing this one! Every effort was made to ensure it is full of as much useful information as possible; please enjoy!

Chapter 1:

The American Woman who Wants to Lose Weight

"The philosophy of fasting calls upon us to know ourselves, to master ourselves, and to discipline ourselves, the better to free ourselves. To fast is to identify our dependencies and free ourselves from them."

- Tariq Ramadan

The desire to lose weight is very common among American women, but it isn't the only thing they want for their bodies. Luckily, intermittent has been proven by research to spur weight loss in American women that were studied, but its health benefits go far beyond weight loss. If you want to feel more energetic, lower your risk of heart disease, and reduce inflammation, intermittent fasting is one lifestyle change that will accomplish all these.

In the four years between 2013 and 2016, half of American citizens said that they wanted to lose weight. This means you are far from the only person in your position. It isn't surprising that more women that were surveyed said they wanted to drop some pounds. While around 60% of women said they had put effort into losing weight, only about 40% of men said the same. Age plays into it too. Just 40% of adults say that they want to lose weight, while 60% of adults under this age say they do. These results from gender and age go across all other demographics: race, income, education, and so on. It has also been found that the more someone weighs, the more likely it is that they say they want to lose weight.

People who want to lose weight employ all sorts of techniques to achieve this end. The most commonly seen techniques are dieting and exercise. As we will see in the book, these two techniques are essential to having success in your health and body. Nowhere in this book will I say that you should not be doing these things.

However, there is a mountain of evidence that the best way to make progress in weight loss is the one that these chapters cover: intermittent fasting in order to trigger autophagy. If you don't believe me, we will continue to cite scientific research backing up this claim. If you need more, you can read through the appendix of studies at the back of the book. The beauty of this technique is that it requires so little change in your day-to-day life when compared to others.

American women have a lot to think about besides losing weight, so a technique that interferes with your life as little as possible is the most practical approach to take. A practical approach like intermittent fasting also makes it more likely that you will continue to follow it through instead of quitting shortly after starting the way that many women do with diet and exercise. If you make exercise your main technique for losing weight, you have to establish a new routine of going to the gym with relative frequency. Of course, all of us could find time in our schedules to do that, but the issue is that changing our schedules so drastically makes us far less likely to keep on track with it. If diet is your main technique, you run into the same obstacle. Your excitement over dieting fades rather quickly once you realize all the planning and calorie counting it demands.

As I will elaborate on later, eating right and exercise are both necessary to some extent to achieve an advanced state of autophagy. They are even more necessary once you get to a certain point in your autophagy journey and become obsessed with triggering it as much as possible. But that will come naturally in the future. For now, you need a plan for losing weight that will work reliably. Intermittent fasting is that plan.

The coming chapters will expand on the definition of intermittent fasting, what benefits you can expect to get from it, and what kinds of intermittent fasting may best suit you. In the meantime, you need to have a basic idea of it to work with.

Intermittent fasting is the practice of going between periods eating ("feasting") and not eating ("fasting"). There are a lot of ways this can be done, but a simple way to start is choosing an amount of time that you will fast every day. You can even start with a number as low as 5 hours and work from there.

An American woman who fasts for 5 hours every day could commit herself not to eat between the hours of 1pm and 6pm every day. After around a month has passed and she has found this to work in her routine, she will want to add a few more hours, making it a 7 hour fast. When this longer one works for another month, she can add more hours to it. A reasonable stretch goal to aim for in the beginning is about 10 to 12 hours. Even with just one small change in your daily eating routine, you can notice surprising changes to your health and body. That is what makes it such a great way of losing weight and unlocking numerous other positive effects on your body.

A Broad Look at How an American Woman Can Lose Weight with Intermittent Fasting

So far, we have explained the reason why intermittent fasting (often shortened to IF) is the perfect solution for you if you want to make your body look and feel healthier.

But in this book, I don't only want to bring IF and autophagy to the general public's attention. I want to our in-depth review of these phenomenally effective lifestyle changes to reach the American woman in particular. If you are an American woman struggling to lose weight, I hope this chapter succeeds in letting you know that *Intermittent Fasting for Women 101* was written for you, especially.

The bulk of our walkthrough on intermittent fasting is going to be about IF itself. However, as effective as IF can surprisingly be on its own, we still have to spend some time discussing diet and exercise, because they too can make a large impact.

Even with IF on our side, there are general guidelines for losing weight that always apply. For one, a woman trying to lose weight will have to take in fewer calories than she is currently. This is just math. A woman who is intermittent fasting consistently but eating the same number of calories in the narrower window of time is not going to find significant success with IF.

Secondly, you have to eat the right foods. You could potentially eat fewer calories than you were before but be getting them from all the wrong places: sugar, saturated fats, and intermittent fasting's biggest enemy: carbs. Instead, you should get your calories from foods that have plenty of important nutrients, vitamins, and minerals. These are foods like fatty fish, whole grains low in carbs, nuts, non-starchy vegetables, some fruit, leafy greens, and more.

We will have plenty of space to go in more detail on which foods to eat in our chapter dedicated to that specifically, but these are your essential foods. Essentially, you want to think about what is really in your food from the standpoint of nutrients. You want to think about how the foods you consume will really affect your body. Once you get used to it, eating healthily is not as cumbersome as you think.

The little things are what matter when it comes to your body and health. For this reason, we still have to dive into the basics of weight loss despite IF being such a reliable method. The first little thing is eating these nutrient-rich foods instead of the nutrient-poor calorie-rich foods you may be used to. The second little thing is getting more exercise. Most American women say they reach their weight goals the most when they follow a consistent routine of diet and exercise, but you should keep in mind that your diet will help you lose weight more than exercise.

Your doctor can help you along your journey to losing weight and answer specific questions that we may not be able to specifically address here. In case you don't visit the doctor soon, you will probably hear the following advice from them: (1) follow the two little things above, (2) get enough sleep every night, and (3) control your level of stress. I do recommend you talk to a doctor when making a lifestyle change like following intermittent fasting, though. Healthy people can make an IF routine without issue the vast majority of the time but talking to a doctor about it can put you at ease.

You are probably cognizant of the fact that different people can use the same methods to lose weight and get very different results. Genes are not the only thing playing a role, though. Everyone burns some calories even when they are not exercising, but the rate at which the calories burn depends on your DNA, the current state of your anatomy, and your health history.

It might help you to keep track of your calories, but perhaps even more important is keeping track of where your calories are coming from. Are they coming from nutrient-rich sources, or from calorie-rich, nutrient-poor sources? One of them will help you lose weight, and the other will hurt you.

Now we need to discuss the matter of how many calories you take in. Logically, you will, of course, lose more weight the fewer calories you consume, but that is not a good thing if you are not eating enough. Doctors say that a woman eating fewer than around 900 calories will hurt you more than help you. Eating fewer calories every day will certainly help you reach your weight goal, but you have to make sure you do it the right way. Not getting enough energy will not only harm your body, but it will not ultimately help you lose weight anyway. If you faint from lack of energy sources, you will lose your self-control and eat a lot in order to get your energy back up, and this will put you back where you started.

As the saying goes, slow and steady wins the race. You should limit your calories at a steady, reasonable amount. Simply consuming as few calories as possible will not help you at all in the long run. It can be tempting when you desperately want to drop several pounds at once, but I strongly urge you not to do this. You can speak with your doctor about how many calories you can safely reduce your daily consumption without running into any health risks. The number they will give you depends on your height, current weight, age, and level of activity.

American women often ask the question: are men better able to lose weight than women? The answer is complicated. It can seem like men have an easier time dropping weight than women, but you have to remember that there are several factors involved. For one, women tend to have a greater share of fat on their bodies compared to muscle, while men tend to have more muscle compared to fat. Since muscle burns more calories than fat, this may be part of the reason that they seem to have an easier time than women.

When you eat, you are in part giving nutrients to your muscles. Men have more muscle on average, so when they eat, more of their calories go to support their muscle. Women, on the other hand, don't have as much muscle to support, so less of their calorie consumption will have this job, and instead, it is more likely to be stored as fat.

Now, I tell everyone, man or woman, that they should try intermittent fasting if they want to lose weight. That said, there are reasons that this works out for women in particular. For instance, one experiment had one group of women lose weight by avoiding unhealthy food, while the other group tried to lose weight by lowering their consumption of calories overall by eating smaller portions. The end result was that the group of women eating fewer calories overall had lower BMIs (body mass indices) by the end of the study.

The same experiment was done on men, and the results were not as strong for them. This suggests that while limiting calories consumed overall could be a better option for women, the kinds of foods consumed may be more important to focus on for men.

As usual, I want to clarify that the specific foods you eat are still very important. Bringing out this scientific study was only meant to serve the purpose of telling you what is more important.

American women should put foods in their bodies that contain the nutrients they need and exercise, but when your main goal is losing weight, the thing you want to focus on most of all is the number of calories consumed. As long as you keep this number at a safe level, you will optimize your success with IF and autophagy.

This is where yet another advantage of IF comes into play. The gains you have from IF are partially from the simple fact of consuming fewer calories. When you don't eat at all during a certain window of the day, this ends up reducing your total number of calories consumed per day. That benefit is only one positive effect of intermittent fasting, although it is a terrific benefit. The most important benefits come from the autophagy triggered by IF. We will have a lot to learn about autophagy in the early chapters.

But on the subject of how an American woman can lose weight, there is still much to consider. We have not even gotten to managing your menstrual cycle while losing weight. While being on your period doesn't make your weight go up or down, it can influence your weight in indirect ways. You will have more of an appetite for sugary and salty food when you have PMS (premenstrual syndrome), as one example. Obviously, eating more foods like these can have quite an effect on your weight, even though your cycle doesn't affect your weight directly. The higher levels of salt in your body can even make your system soak up more water instead of disposing of it, giving you more water weight. These ways that your cycle makes losing weight harder can be especially troublesome as an American woman, where sugary and salty foods are widespread and cheap. Your best bet for resisting these temptations is not buying them in the first place. Fill your pantry and fridge with nutrient-rich foods; don't put the sugary and salty foods there to begin with.

The same way your period can indirectly affect your weight, your weight can affect your period as well. Although our end goal is to lose weight, losing weight or gaining weight in a short span of time can have consequences for your menstrual cycle. Your period may not come on time or may not come at all. Many women with weight problems like obesity have this issue. On the other hand, if your period is coming on schedule on a regular basis, this is a good indicator of overall health. Accomplishing your goal weight will help make your period come at a regular schedule.

Trying to lose weight can also become a challenge after menopause. For example, on average menopausal women put on 5 pounds. Estrogen actually helps regulate your weight, so the fact that your estrogen levels are lower may be part of the reason it is harder to lose weight or maintain your weight. But we can't only blame it on menopause. Oftentimes, gaining weight at this stage in life can be due to a slowed metabolism that comes with age in general, eating too many unhealthy foods and not enough healthy ones, and not getting enough exercise.

We also lose significant muscle mass with age. With less muscle mass comes fewer calories than our bodies use, and therefore convert to fat. All of these facts about losing weight on menopause should teach us to do the same two little things that all American women should do to lose weight: keep up an active lifestyle and eat healthful foods.

If you are an American woman over the age of 50, I also recommend that you don't eat as many calories that you used to when you were younger. There are two main reasons for this: (1) women don't need as many calories as men because of having less muscle mass, more fat, and being smaller in size in general, and (2) women over 50 tend to expend less energy than they used to, so they don't need as many calories in the first place.

If you fall into the demographic of women over 50, you should speak with your doctor about how many calories you can safely limit your diet to lose weight. Their answer may surprise you because women generally don't need as many calories when they are older.

Intermittent Fasting as an Alternative to Less Healthy Methods that May Not Even Work

When American women try to lose weight, they have many options with which to approach the situation. Unfortunately, many of them will only help you lose weight that you will put back on the moment you get back into your normal routine. Not only that, but they can have negative health consequences.

It is astonishing how many doctors now recommend weight-loss prescriptions to menopausal women. Usually, they will only do this if you have a BMI over 30 (if you are obese) or if you are overweight and you are looking at other health risks because of your weight as determined by hypertension or high cholesterol. Additionally, a good doctor will make sure you have tried the two little things we mentioned earlier before prescribing you medicine: regular exercise and dieting. They will normally only prescribe it to you if you have not seen results from these methods. While it is understandable to want to avoid the health risks of being overweight or obese, the side effects that accompany these medicines may outweigh the benefits. They include migraines, coughing, tiredness, constipation, and even dissociation.

Again, it makes complete sense that a doctor might prescribe these medications to women so they can lose weight and can be at lower risk for diseases related to weight. But it is not necessary for you to take these measures and accept these side effects, because you can do intermittent fasting instead. IF has no side effects — only good ones, like triggering autophagy and losing weight. Much like taking a pill, IF doesn't require much change in your daily life. It only requires that you *don't* do something during a small window of your day: eat.

Many American women are choosing intermittent fasting over medication because of it. You can join them today. These upcoming chapters equip you with all the information you need to do IF successfully so you can enjoy its effects on your body and health.

Chapter 2:

What is Intermittent Fasting?

"The best of all medicines is resting and fasting."

- Benjamin Franklin

Fasting has become a hot topic as of late. The buzz around intermittent fasting, in particular, opened a door for many women who wanted to lose weight but were worried about the heavy commitment of a day-long water-only fast. It's hard to say exactly what intermittent fasting is because there are a variety of ways to go about it. When you do an intermittent fast, you are going back and forth in a regular cycle between fasting and eating normally. I will cover all types of IF (the abbreviation for intermittent fasting) in this book, and you can decide which best suits your stage in life and goals.

Many women have seen real change happen in their health, thanks to IF. You could join them by following the various tips contained here. The first task we have to complete is giving you a broad overview of all things intermittent fasting: what the benefits are, what the science says, what different kinds of intermittent fasting exist, and what foods you should eat when you intermittent fast.

We can start with the health benefits. Women who follow a routine of intermittent fasting feel that they have more energy, burn more fat, and lower their chances of getting diabetes or heart disease. Researchers looking into IF find that its practitioners have higher success rates than people who do extended, interrupted fasts and people who use exercise as their chief method to lose weight. They suggest the success of IF is because it can be woven seamlessly into the participants' lives without their having to change multiple aspects of their normal routines.

Intermittent fasting eliminates the perfectionism that sometimes ruins other weight loss techniques. IF doesn't ask that you constantly pay attention to the number of calories you consume. It doesn't punish you harshly for falling out of it for one day.

We will learn more about the science underlying IF later on but suffice to say that you can earn the positive health effects of autophagy without doing extended fasts. The experiments studying people doing IF consistently demonstrate that they see good results from only doing IF, without doing more demanding fasts such as extended water fasting.

In the last chapter, we talked about the study showing that women have more success in losing weight by reducing caloric intake compared to when they pay close attention to what they are eating. This is precisely what IF entails. Nutrition is still important, which is why we still have a chapter on it, but regardless of what you eat, you will still see some amount of positive change from IF.

I hope that I have at least made you curious about getting these results from IF in your own life — and to do that, you will need to find a way to implement IF in a way that works for you. It's time to answer the question directly: in the simplest terms, what do I have to do to start intermittent fasting today? What is required of me to start seeing these effects on my health?

Because of the nature of IF, you will, unfortunately, have to start tomorrow, not today — unless it is morning right now. Ask yourself how many hours you think you can fast tomorrow. Let's say it is 6 hours. Most people start their fast after lunch and break it for dinner. Keep in mind that you will have to eat lunch relatively early so that you do not have dinner too late. If you have dinner too late, your system will take hours to start up autophagy while you sleep because you will still be digesting food. You should be able to see now why many women find they are able to succeed in losing weight with IF when they were not successful using other methods. What I described in the last paragraph is all that IF amounts to on your end.

Of course, practice is always harder than theory. I will never tell you that intermittent fasting takes no willpower and resistance on your end. Compared to other potential options, though, IF is extremely straightforward. Still, you might have a long way to go to be ready to live by IF. Maybe you still need to be convinced by the number of studies that we will cover proving the health benefits. Maybe you are scientifically minded and need to learn more about autophagy.

You might get inspired when I tell you all the delicious foods you can eat when you intermittent fast to make autophagy even stronger; you might be ready to start after you read about all the different kinds of IF, and you find the one that is perfect for you.

The chapters after this one will explore these topics and more. This one will give you a general idea of all of them so you can keep reading with an informed picture of what you are getting into. You may even choose to check the Table of Contents and read the chapters that interest you the most first. It is your choice. Just be sure to read through all of them at some point, so you don't miss any important knowledge.

Intermittent Fasting: Looking at its Effects on Health More Closely

In few words, IF helps you lose weight using short-term and long-term strategies, by depriving your system of calories so you accumulate less fat in the short term and by detoxifying your cells in the long term through autophagy. The short-term strategy is what tends to draw women in, but the long-term strategy is what makes IF great for your body overall.

This is not the same kind of detox that you may be sick of hearing about online. The autophagy triggered by IF is a detox that has always existed in biology and can simply be jumpstarted naturally by fasting. While a detox like "juicing" will claim to clean out your system, supporters of juice diets have no data to back up this assertion. Meanwhile, autophagy has been studied by scientists and nutritionists for decades now. We know that it works to lose weight. We know that it does so without hurting your body the way that other methods do — not only does it not hurt your body, but it has long-term positive consequences like less inflammation and lower cholesterol.

Every organism on the planet goes through autophagy, so you are not even putting your body through anything strange to get these effects on your health. If you had never heard of the word autophagy before, it would still occur in your body. By learning how to trigger autophagy through intermittent fasting, you are simply learning how to optimize it. Autophagy doesn't involve any strange medicines or foods. Whatever you put into your body; you can still trigger autophagy with IF.

Of course, your diet does affect how powerful your autophagy is, but we will talk about that in a moment. For now, I want to tell you more about the short-term effects of IF. The first we will explore is the enhanced health of your skin. The first layer of skin that you have is called the epidermis. You see your epidermis every day because this is the visible part of your skin. There are layers of skin below it, but you don't see those layers unless you suffer an injury. We will go into more scientific detail on the process of autophagy in the section after this one, but you will need a crash course to understand why autophagy triggered by IF is so good for your skin, and your epidermis in specific.

Both parts of the English word "autophagy" are of Greek origin. "Auto" has the meaning "self" (which you might already know) and "phagy" has the meaning "eat." Put the two together, and you get the fundamental concept of autophagy. Your cells "eat themselves" when they are under acute stress. Unlike you, your cells need energy constantly — even when you are sleeping. They will get it from whatever source they can find. Even when you are not putting food into your body (even when you are fasting), your cells find ways of getting energy. When in this state of stress, their main sources of energy are the following: cell organelles that stopped working, proteins that are no longer being used, and toxins that came from outside your body.

For your first fast, you will notice big changes in your body after only a day. These drastic changes are thanks to autophagy. I guarantee you the first change you will notice is in your skin. It will remind you of when you were younger because of its newfound elasticity and glow. These improvements in your skin are because of autophagy. On an invisible level of your skin pores, your skin cells are cleaning out the toxins described above. On the massive scale of your whole pore, that makes a huge difference. The autophagy results in skin that isn't filled with cellular waste.

The cleaning out of cellular waste isn't the only reason your skin gets better. It's also because you have an increase in the collagen protein in your skin. Collagen is a protein that your skin cells make more of when you are younger. Collagen is the reason the skin of younger people looks the way it is. As you get older, your skin cells make less collagen because they are less effective. This is where autophagy changes everything. Autophagy does two things to make new, young cells: (1) builds them from scratch using the raw materials obtained from eating their own cellular waste or (2) renovates existing cells with new organelles constructed with raw materials obtained from eating their own cellular waste.

Everything should be coming together with intermittent fasting and autophagy now. It all goes like this: you do even a moderate level of fasting that increases your autophagy and then when your skin cells go through autophagy, they make younger cells or make existing cells like younger cells.

The best part is that the improved health of your skin is only the beginning. The main reason everyone who does IF does it is because they want to lose weight. Fasting proves time and time again that it is the best way of doing it. This point has already been driven home, so I will add just one extra point to it: you won't just lose weight, but you will be able to relax about loose skin as well.

The infamous "skin curtain" is the excess skin that people are afraid of getting when they lose weight. It is astonishing how many people say they don't want to lose weight out of fear of loose skin. The good news is that autophagy comes to the rescue on this front. By losing weight through fasting, you cut down on calories and trigger autophagy at the same time. Autophagy's job is to break down poorly performing cells and replace them with new, young cells, or at least replace their organelles with new ones. That's why people who lose weight through fasting are proven to deal with far fewer issues with loose skin. Not only do they have less loose skin to deal with in the beginning, but they are better able to manage what loose skin they do have because of the better health of their skin.

I told you that you would have more energy when you did intermittent fasting, and now it's time to explain the scientific reason why. Autophagy is behind it, as usual. Maybe you have already deduced why by now. The short answer is that the autophagy that IF triggers makes your cells more efficient, and more efficient cells means more energy for you.

As you get older, your cells are less effective than they used to be. They are littered with cellular waste and their cell organs (organelles) are damaged and ineffective in themselves. Autophagy is the remedy to this problem. Autophagy disposes of organelles that aren't performing optimally and disposes of cellular waste and misfolded proteins that are taking up space in your cells without doing anything useful. When all of your cells go through autophagy regularly and take care of these issues, you have more energy because your cells make up all of you, and that makes your system more efficient with energy overall.

Now let's go in more detail on the long-term positive health effects of autophagy triggered through intermittent fasting.

There is research showing that autophagy will fight against tumors, and there is also research showing that it will help them grow — only because cancer cells are cells, too. But although autophagy can work on both sides, the important thing is that autophagy promotes the health of your non-cancerous cells, which will always outnumber your cancerous ones in the early stages. Of course, most people triggering autophagy are doing it to prevent cancer in the early stages and not to stop cancer that is already progressing, so this is all they need. Intermittent fasting has been found to be a powerful tool in combating cancer. While cancer, in general, is still under debate as something that autophagy can prevent altogether, the jury is no longer out for Alzheimer's disease, Parkinson's disease, and Huntington's Disease. We know that these are preventable with autophagy now. Autophagy has been proven to be incredibly effective for matters of the brain.

For long-term problems especially, autophagy is a powerful tool for ensuring the viability and survivability of cells. Scientists did not see autophagy as such a big actor for these diseases until recently. This discovery changes everything scientists thought they knew about the biological process. Excitingly, as I keep telling you, you can trigger autophagy yourself through intermittent fasting.

But cancer is far from the only age-related condition that autophagy can address. Diseases of the mind, heart disease, diseases related to autoimmune failure, and more can be helped with autophagy. While we still aren't sure if autophagy can stop tumors from continuing to grow altogether once they reach a certain size, we know that they can keep the rest of your body around the tumor healthy. This can only be a good thing for fighting cancer, and its why autophagy is useful in preventing all these other diseases too.

In diabetic people, there are clusters of protein built up in their arteries. When they use intermittent fasting to trigger autophagy, scientists can see that these protein clusters are cleared out.

Sometimes books about the newest findings in science with regard to health can be misleading about what the scientific consensus is, but I want this one to be clear about what all scientists agree on. This way, it is as useful and truthful to women as possible.

We know for sure that autophagy is a main player — if not *the* main player — in fighting against neurodegenerative diseases like Huntington's, Alzheimer's, and Parkinson's. It plays this role by cleaning out the build-ups of proteins that happen in your neurons, leading to clogging and brain dysfunction.

Scientists even agree about what causes these protein buildups in the first place, at this point. As your autophagy occurs in the brain, a special organelle called the autophagosome binds with your lysosome (your cell stomach). In many cases of autophagy, this is the normal way that it occurs. Your autophagosome binds with your lysosome in order to break down the cellular waste.

However, what causes the protein buildups is the abnormally strong bond that the autophagosome has with the lysosome. This strong bond between the autophagosome and the lysosome causes what biologists call a "clogging effect." The clogging effect makes your proteins build up in your neurons, leading to neurodegeneration.

You can read more about the details of this science soon enough, but these are the basics of what causes these diseases. As you can see, autophagy is at the very center of it. If you want to prevent these diseases — as everyone does — you have to trigger autophagy as much as possible, so your cells clean out your proteins.

You might think this sounds counterintuitive since these buildups happen in the first place because of autophagy occurring and the autophagosome binding too tightly with the lysosome. But this abnormal binding is only an issue when your autophagy is occurring at a maintenance level. Scientists who study autophagy say that your autophagy is in "maintenance mode" when it is happening at a low level, just as it always does. You see, autophagy is always happening in your body somewhere, but that does not mean it is happening at a significant level.

Your autophagosome and lysosome can cause the "clogging effect" when your autophagy only happens in maintenance mode and you do not trigger advanced autophagy to clean out the resulting protein buildup. All you have to do to clear out this protein build up is do intermittent fasting, trigger advanced autophagy, and prevent the protein buildup that could cause you to go through neurodegeneration. If you want to know more about the biology of this process or about the link between neurodegenerative diseases and autophagy, you will have plenty to look forward to in the coming chapters. For now, we will continue outlining the long-term benefits of using IF to trigger autophagy.

We listed losing weight as a short-term effect, which it is — but it is also a long-term benefit. People who are overweight or obese have higher risk of heart disease, diabetes, and failing autoimmune systems. When you lose weight, you lower your risk of all these problems.

Therefore, you should also consider it to have a long-term positive effect on your health.

While this won't apply to every woman's situation, there has also been testing on the effects of autophagy on people going through chemotherapy for cancer. The researchers looked at a group going through therapy without fasting and a group who did intermittent fasting during the chemotherapy.

The group that fasted while going through chemotherapy had significantly lower amounts of dead white blood cells in their systems. If you don't know already, chemotherapy has some negative side effects when it kills cancer cells, and one of them is killing good cells like white blood cells.

White blood cells do a very important job when they are alive, but like every other cell, they become toxic when they die. Unfortunately, chemotherapy tends to kill a lot of white blood cells in the process of killing cancer cells.

That's where autophagy comes in. The patients who fasted during chemotherapy had significantly less dead white blood cells creating toxins in their bodies because intermittent fasting got rid of them. Intermittent fasting led their bodies to seek nutrients from inside the body;

there were a lot of dead white blood cells in their body, so autophagy took care of those. As a result, they did not have all these dead cells polluting their bodies.

There is a lot of research about the effect of autophagy triggered by fasting on people with cancer. Another study looked at women with breast cancer who did a fast lasting 12 hours daily. These women did not see their cancer return as often as women who did not fast. This means that not only does autophagy have implications for lessening the side effects of common cancer treatment likes chemotherapy, but it can even lower the chances that your cancer will come back once it goes.

We are still waiting to see if pharmacists can manage to create a medicine that will take advantage of the power of autophagy. There are supplements that claim to trigger autophagy, but none of those claims are substantial at the moment, so your best option is to focus on making autophagy happen through intermittent fasting. But it is possible that, one day, scientists will use their knowledge on autophagy to create a medicine that cures diseases like Alzheimer's and cancer. The possibilities are endless for autophagy.

As far as long-term benefits of autophagy go, it has even been shown to lower the amount of inflammation in your body. When you have less inflammation in your body, your DNA in your cells is far less likely to be damaged. Damaged DNA and high inflammation are big risk factors for diseases like cancer, so these are highly important long-term effects. When parts of your body are inflamed, autophagy does its part by taking care of these damages. Once these damages have been taken care of, you can make new parts that are newer, younger, and less vulnerable to damage. It has even been shown that mice who were bred in a lab who went through autophagy triggered through fasting had lower rates of cancer than rats who did not fast. The ones who did not trigger autophagy had higher rates of cancer.

Your digestive health is surprisingly important to your long-term health outcomes, and autophagy can help in keeping this part of your body healthy as well. It is so important because the parts of your body that control your digestive system are constantly working — they never stop. When they give your digestive system a break by fasting, you are giving it time to stop what it is doing and do repairs. Your tissues in your digestive system have the opportunity to clear out cellular waste and make their systems more efficient at the cellular level.

This makes this system of your body more efficient, all because you are able to trigger autophagy to keep it clean. People often underestimate the importance of their gut health, but it is actually one of the parts of your body you should protect the most. If you are not able to get nutrients with a healthy gut, none of the other systems in your body are able to work the way they should.

We would be remiss to forget about your autoimmune system in the context of autophagy. Your autoimmune system is the way your body attack infections and disease. It fights cancer before it can grow to the size of a tumor. But it isn't only about cancer: your autoimmune system keeps any infection from turning into a disease.

Doctors now say that preventive medicine is the most important kind of medicine, and your autoimmune system is the main player in your body's natural disease preventive mechanism. When you do intermittent fasting, you keep this vital system healthy and prevent age-related disease. This is a good place to start when describing all the good things autophagy can do for your body by simply limiting the window of time that you are eating every day. However, if you want to get the short-term and long-term effects, you have to keep a few things in mind.

First of all, you can't expect to get these results by simply fasting every once in a while. If you eat poorly, drink a lot, smoke, get little sleep, or have any number of habits that are bad for your health, you can't expect to do intermittent fasting and have it repair all the damage you do to your body from these habits. Successfully triggering autophagy with intermittent fasting requires that you are at least somewhat healthy in other areas of your habits as well. Autophagy needs your body to maintain some level of basic health in order to do its job. It can't do that job without your help.

There is not enough space in this book to tell you how to stop all of these bad habits, but I will do our best to consider the lifestyle of the average American woman when helping you get intermittent fasting into your life.

Intermittent Fasting and Autophagy

Autophagy is the natural way your body disposes of toxic chemicals in your cells. You can't see it happening without a microscope, but your cells have been going through autophagy for your entire life without you ever noticing. In just the last twenty years, scientists have learned much about the metabolic process of autophagy. Most importantly for our purposes, they have learned more and more about how autophagy's implications for fighting against disease and aging.

The entire foundation of using intermittent fasting for losing weight and getting healthier is our current scientific understanding of autophagy. We know for a fact that autophagy can help us attain better general health and live longer. Autophagy isn't just for losing weight, however — although it does that job better than any other method. It used to be that people went through autophagy quite often. We went through autophagy more back in the days before industrial agriculture because we did not expect to have food all the time.

Nowadays in the industrialized world, most people rarely miss a meal. We always have food around us. But people back in the day did not even have an expectation to eat every single day. Our bodies went through advanced autophagy very regularly because of this. We can even say that our bodies are more built for not eating every day than they are for eating constantly as we do right now.

Our first encounter with autophagy in the world of science was thanks to the French scientist named Christian De Duve. He and a group of biologists took note of a bizarre organelle that they had never seen before; they named it the lysosome.

Before we knew all that we know now about autophagy, scientists thought that the lysosome was simply an organelle made for disposing of garbage. If you think about it, this doesn't even make logical sense, because there is not really such thing as disposing of something. You can change the form of something, but not dispose of it. If the lysosome were really an organelle that just kept breaking things down without recycling those parts, then eventually those tiny waste particles would build-up with nowhere to go.

Now we have an explanation for this problem because of autophagy, and this explanation has important takeaways for doctors, biologists, and anyone who cares about their health.

The Japanese scientist Yoshinori Ohsumi was the first scientist to get deeply interested in the lysosome of yeast cells. 2016 was the year he won the Nobel Prize when he learned that the lysosome was the center of a cellular process called autophagy. His key finding was that our cells never "dispose of" anything — they simply break down cellular waste into raw materials, and then use these materials to build new structures.

Ohsumi has created a new definition of autophagy. He says that autophagy is the way our cells break down waste materials for the purpose of freeing up space, killing harmful foreign toxins, and creating raw materials that can be used for building new cells. When Ohsumi first started, he was the first scientist to really have any interest in this topic. He started a scientific movement around autophagy when his research uncovered all the implications that autophagy has for our bodies. Not only did Ohsumi uncover much of our modern understanding of autophagy, but he was the one who coined the phrase "cell recycling." Cell recycling is what happens once autophagy is finished.

When your cells have cleaned themselves out, they use these raw materials for constructing things that other cells can use. They can also use these raw materials to create new cells if there is enough.

Now we know that autophagy can be considered the most important process for your cells both individually and collectively. Autophagy matters to your cells individually because it keeps them alive as well as possible; it matters collectively because your cells have to work together to be useful to your body as a whole, and autophagy keeps them working together smoothly when the process keeps them repaired and "cleaned out."

We will have an entire chapter dedicated to the science that makes intermittent fasting such a great way of keeping your system in great shape. For now, this should provide you with all you need to know to continue on with a solid understanding of the underlying process of autophagy making your fasting worth it.

You also need to keep in mind the times that you should be eating these foods. The whole purpose of autophagy is lost if you eat during the times you are supposed to fast. That's because consuming anything puts your digestive system at work. When your body digests food, your autophagy stops. You need to really make sure you are not eating at all during these times that you have designated to be your fasting windows.

Even eating 20 calories disrupts autophagy entirely. You may think that eating a banana or a small snack during your fasting window won't change anything, but that isn't true at all. You would be shocked at how much changes in your body when you put food into it. The fact that so much changes is the reason why autophagy is so potent in the first place — because it is recovering from all the times that you were putting food into your body.

The Ideal Diet for a Woman Doing Intermittent Fasting

Before we dive into the subject of what you eat when you fast, I need to issue a warning to you: there are people selling supplements that they say will trigger autophagy. At the moment, no such supplements exist. That means you need to be wary of claims like these. There are scientists trying to create a medication with this effect, but it has not been made yet.

The first important vitamin is also the easiest one to get into your body: Vitamin D. This is an essential vitamin to a myriad of biological processes that your system goes through, and autophagy is one of them — so if you don't have enough Vitamin D, you won't be able to get the autophagy that you need.

You don't ever want to think about diet as your only means of triggering autophagy. Everything needs to be in place to some extent: you need to keep up a diet of nutrient-rich foods, exercise, get plenty of sleep, avoid unhealthy habits, and fast. The great thing about doing more for autophagy through diet is that it focuses certain organs in your body to make sure you are getting autophagy where you need it.

We will start with ginger as an example to illustrate this. Ginger contains a chemical called 6-shogaol, which actually slows the growth of cells in your lungs. It probably seems counterproductive to ingest something that stops your cells from growing when you are trying to prevent cancer or some other lung disease. However, ginger is an excellent complement to autophagy because this chemical suppresses cell growth.

6-shogaol suppresses all cell growth, meaning that even cancer cells will not be able to grow as well when you add this chemical into your system.

Omega-3 fats are probably something that you have heard of before. They are considered a "healthy fat," a kind of fat that your body needs for autophagy. People who get plenty of these healthy fats into their bodies have been shown to have more advanced autophagy than people who do not. Autophagy is greatly aided by unsaturated fats like Omega-3 fats.

With that in mind, you should know that with Omega-3 fats and all of the nutrients we mention, you need to make a real effort to get them from your regular diet rather than from supplements. For example, the effectiveness of Omega-3 fats in making people's bodies healthier and supporting autophagy are scientifically substantiated, but it has only been tested in people who got them from real food like fish. There is no backing to the idea that the Omega-3 fats that some people get some supplements are going to give you this same effect.

Getting your Omega-3 fats from a supermarket is not your best option, either. Grocery stores these days are known to get their meats from factory farms. Meat coming from factory farms does not have Omega-3 fats because of what factory farms feed their cattle. Instead of eating grass or other natural foods, they consume a lot of chemicals. Instead of indirectly getting the Omega-

3 fats from grass through your meat, you are indirectly getting whatever chemical foods these factory farms give to their animals.

It goes without saying that you need to eat plenty of vegetables when you are doing intermittent fasting, too. It is a simple fact that a lot of people don't like vegetables at all, but thankfully there are ways of getting around this. One of them is putting your vegetables in a blender together with some fruit. If you get your vegetables this way, you should remember not to add too much fruit into the blender. While fruits are good for us, they have a lot of natural sugar in them, which is still bad for us in large quantities just like artificial sugars.

The next thing you should consider consuming to help in autophagy and IF is green tea. The chemical in green tea that you are really looking for triggers AMPK, which is an enzyme in your system that boosts the effectiveness of autophagy. Green tea goes best with turmeric, because they both help with autophagy.

Next, you should find somewhere that you can start picking up the reishi mushroom and eating it on the regular. The reishi mushroom is a special case because it can significantly slow the growth of one cell in particular:

cancer cells in the colon. The colon is a very common place to start seeing cancer, so the reishi mushroom is really something that you should consider adding to your diet. It works by helping the growth of non-cancer cells when cancer cells are growing in the colon. When non-cancer cells are able to grow and flourish in your body alongside cancer cells, this really helps keep cancer at bay and fight it. Each cell does its part in trying to overwhelm the cancer cells. Normally, the cancer cells in the colon will actively try to stop the non-cancer cells from growing, and the chemicals in the reishi mushroom does their part in keeping this from occurring.

Looking at autophagy and intermittent fasting from the perspective of diet can be very inspiring because you can look at them from more than one point of view. You feel as though you are triggering autophagy in every way possible from the simple action of eating certain foods that you know for sure are helping your autophagy.

Good practitioners of autophagy and intermittent fasting will use several methods to make their autophagy as strong as possible. I have done extensive research about what scientists say on these different diets, and I am only recommending foods to you that are proved to work.

If you are still having issues deciding which method of triggering autophagy is right for you, looking at the foods you eat might be a good place to start. This book strongly recommends intermittent fasting since it is known to be the most consistent way of getting more autophagy to happen in your system, but everyone is different, so you might want to think about all of your options.

You also need to think about what not to eat when you are thinking about autophagy. Our number one enemy against autophagy is carbs. Everyone knows about the bad reputation that carbs have, but not enough know exactly why we should lessen how many carbs we put into our bodies. Did you know that the average American gets nearly 60% of their calories every day from carbs? It seems incredible, but it's true. Not only do American women have the issue of eating a lot of calories without a plan to burn them off with exercise, but they are getting many of these calories from a source that is notoriously difficult for your system to break down.

Here is the true reason that makes carbs so dangerous for someone trying to lose weight, especially for someone who has a plan to do intermittent fasting: when your gut is holding all of your foods and breaking them down, it has proteins, fats, and carbohydrates. No matter how much fat and protein it has to break down, no matter what other factors are at play, your body will always break down carbs first.

This is because the very nature of carbohydrates makes them extremely challenging to break down. Therefore, your stomach will decide to work on them last. This is why you need to choose a diet that is very low in carbs if you want to succeed in intermittent fasting. Your new life as a slimmer, healthier, and more youthful woman may even depend upon you eating fewer carbs. You will be surprised how many times a day carbs make their way into your diet. This will seriously impair your autophagy. Another way of illustrating this is by looking at how much it reduces your autophagy.

We can use an example where you finish eating a meal at 1pm and then stop eating until 9pm. This seems like an 8-hour fast. However, it really is a 4-hour fast. This is because when you stop eating at 1pm, it takes your body 4 hours to digest your food. You aren't done digesting it until 5pm, and then you start eating again at 9pm. Thus, your fast was really 4 hours long. Now, let's put carbohydrates into the picture. Let's say the last meal you eat before you start fasting is a bowl filled with pasta at 1pm. Then you don't eat again until 9pm. Take a guess at how long of a fast this really was.

The answer is 0 hours. That's right: it takes 8 hours for your body to digest carbs. Even though you stop eating for 8 hours after the bowl of pasta, your stomach is just now finishing digesting the carbs from the pasta at 9pm, and then you are just putting more food into your body again, stopping autophagy. Your autophagy depends heavily on what you are consuming. It relies on you getting plenty of healthy fats and not eating too many carbs. Practically speaking, most people doing IF to lose weight should reduce their consumption of carbs to be as low as possible.

Now, we need to spend some time talking about fats. It can be confusing because a lot of people are under the impression that fats are bad overall. They don't realize how much their bodies rely on fats to perform basic functions — including autophagy. Not all fats are the same, however. Because of the chemical composition of different fats, some of them are essential, while some of them should be limited to being eaten as little as possible. The fats in your diet can be the hardest thing for you to control, and the way it works can be hard to understand. They can be some of the best things for your body and some of the worst things for your body. First, we will get into what can make them good when you eat the right ones.

Firstly, your system depends on fats because they are one of its sources of energy. Fats can even store vitamins and minerals. Fats are essential for building membranes around your cells and sheaths around your nerves. On a bigger scale, you have fat for moving your muscles, clotting your blood, and keeping your inflammation at normal levels. Generally, we can say that your saturated fats are bad for you, and your unsaturated fats are good for you. Trans fats are especially bad for you, but you don't have to think about that too much, because now they are banned in most places.

Trans fats are a great demonstration of what can make your fats bad. These kinds of fats only come into being because of the industrial, artificial processes that create and preserve food these days. They have no use in your body and can only harm you. This is the reason that they are not allowed in the United States anymore.

Then you have saturated fats. Doctors say that you should be keeping your level of saturated fats to less than

10 percent of all your calories. If at all possible, don't eat saturated fats when you have them as an option.

Meanwhile, doctors want us to get about 30 percent of our calories from good fats. To a lot of people, this seems like a lot of fats for doctors to recommend to us! It goes to show you how different kinds of fats have such different effects on our bodies.

We have plenty more to discuss in the chapter coming later about what foods to eat when doing IF, but this should give you a good preview on what to expect later. Now you can read about what different options you have for methods of IF.

Your Options for Different Methods of Intermittent Fasting

If none of the methods of intermittent fasting discussed thus far appeal to you, this is a section that *will* appeal to you. We will discuss these methods more and hopefully convince you that there is one that suits your needs.

I will start by telling you that intermittent fasting is by far the most popular way to fast overall. Outside of intermittent fasting, the only other legitimate option is called extended water fasting. Extended water fasting, usually just called water fasting, is when you only consume water for a period of time, usually lasting 24 hours or longer. We will get into water fasting a little bit in this book, but there are many reasons that we will mostly stick to intermittent fasting.

I say that the non-intermittent fasts outside of water fasting are not legitimate simply because there is no research supporting their claims the way there is for water fasting and intermittent fasting. We will start by talking about what other fasts you may hear about, and I will tell you why you can forget about them entirely, because either they won't work to help you lose weight, they are bad for your body, or oftentimes, both. The most dangerous one is called dry fasting. Dry fasting is the same thing as water fasting, but you don't even consume water. It is hard to say why this idea even exists because there is no reason to believe that it would be more effective in helping you lose weight than water fasting. Sure, you will lose water weight for a temporary span of time, but then you will go back to drinking water and gain it all back again. It does not even keep the water weight off of you.

But all of that is beside the point; you don't want to lose water weight. Hydration is one of the most important things to be mindful of when caring for your body, and when it gets too low, that is bad for you in general — not to mention bad for your autophagy. I said to watch your diet, exercise, fasting, and sleep when you want to trigger autophagy, but you have to watch your water consumption, too. Not having any water for your cells dries them out and prevents them from working the way that they should.

Once you get a grip on the intermittent fasting stuff, you might want to dip your toes into water fasting. The best way to do this is by participating in the 24-hour fast.

When you do a true, traditional fast, you don't eat at all for at least a day. This is the essence of the water fast, too, but extended water fasting can last for multiple days. With the 24-hour fast, you are only dedicating yourself to fasting for 24 hours. This is a lot easier than you might think.

Next, we have what is known as consecutive day fasting. Maybe fasting for a set number of hours every single day sounds like a commitment that you won't be able to keep up. If that's the case, consecutive day fasting might be right for you. You might decide on fasting for 12 hours every other day instead of 8 hours every single day. This way, your fasts balance each other out. Another advantage of the consecutive day fast is you have something to look forward to on your fasting days. You know that you will not have to fast the next day; this can be very motivating for a lot of people.

When it comes to fasts that you should avoid, we could talk about protein fasting. Protein fasting is when protein is the only thing that you consume. Protein may be an important thing for you to get into your system, but it is definitely not wise to make it the only nutrient you get. In fact, it is best for you to eat a pretty low amount of protein. Your body will break down fat before protein, and as a result, your autophagy will be better if you don't eat as much of it. The logic behind protein fasting simply doesn't hold up, so you shouldn't pay any attention to it.

In truth, at the end of the day, this is your body that we are talking about, so the way you choose to fast is your decision alone. You will always have the freedom to tailor your fast any way you want. As long as you follow the guidance in our book, you can do fasting your own way.

Chapter 3:
Benefits of Intermittent Fasting

There is no longer a debate on this point: intermittent fasting has many significant and positive consequences for your health. People who have it as part of their routine say their minds feel clearer, and they are capable of more productive work because their bodies have more energy. They report an increase in muscle and a decrease in body fat. Insulin goes down, your skin gets shinier and more elastic, and your heart is healthier. And all these benefits came from, when you really break it down, simply skipping a meal or two a day.

We just summarized many of these positive health effects in the previous chapter, but in Chapter 3, we have the opportunity to provide you with even more knowledge about how intermittent fasting will improve your body's health.

Autophagy: Nature's Detoxifier

Now that you have learned the science underlying the benefits of autophagy, we can dive deeper into the cleansing side of autophagy. The science behind autophagy is what makes intermittent fasting better than other strategies to increase your health that end up doing more harm than good. It tells us that autophagy is something that all of us should be thinking about — even if we are not trying to lose weight — because it just has that much influence on our bodies.

Even as you read into the third chapter, I can guarantee you that you have not yet scratched the surface of what autophagy will do for your body once you find yourself doing it every day. Look at it this way: there is definitely a lot of evidence that kale is a superfood that is very good for you since it is filled with so many vitamins and nutrients that your body needs. That's why everyone says that you should eat it.

Some people take scientific facts, like kale being good for you, and twist them to make it seem like kale is the only food you should be eating. They try to sell you diets based on blending kale and drinking it throughout the day. While it's true that consuming more kale would be good for you, kale still doesn't compare to autophagy. That's because while kale is great, it still doesn't give you everything you need, and more importantly, it isn't literally essential to your body.

On the other hand, autophagy is essential to your body. It happens whether you like it or not, and if you never thought about autophagy in your whole life, it would still happen. If your cells didn't go through autophagy, your cells would die, and you would die along with them. This is what makes detoxifying your body with autophagy different from detoxifying your body with something like kale. We are taking something that your body already does and needs and maximizing it to its greatest potential.

No matter how much energy you feel like you are using at any given time, your cells are always using energy. Unlike you and me, they do not get to sleep and recover from a long day. This is what makes autophagy a central part of a cell's functions: when you fast and your cells' food resources are depleted, they still need energy to keep on going — so they find their energy in the nooks and crannies. Your cells eat their own unused proteins, broken organelles, and their autophagosomes start working extra hard to find the toxins that are in various parts of your system. They are extra motivated to do this when you fast because if they don't, they can't keep doing the things that cells do.

Our cells don't care about their state of cleanliness the way you do. You care about their cleanliness because they work much better when they have cleared out the toxins, and that's where all the positive health effects of autophagy come from. But since your cells don't care themselves, they will let things get very crowded: they will have toxins all over and will simply die off when it becomes so much that they can't work properly.

Of course, they will eventually go through some maintenance mode autophagy when you go to sleep. But you are reading this book because you want your cells to go above and beyond what they would do normally — because that is what is going to get the best health outcomes for you.

We really let our cells make a mess of themselves in the modern-day. Once you do your first intermittent fast, you will realize how much we eat every day like it's nothing. To briefly look at things from a philosophical standpoint, we are always filling ourselves with stuff, and we don't give ourselves a chance to empty ourselves out. Autophagy comes in for that last part. Our bodies are not anywhere equipped to deal with all the junk we stuff into our bodies these days, so we have to think about our cells proactively and make sure they use autophagy to keep things running efficiently.

We all know the artificial chemicals that inevitably end up in our bodies in today's society. If we don't deliberatively take care of it by doing intermittent fasting, some of these may end up having negative long-term consequences on our health. I don't advocate for being paranoid about what chemicals are in our foods, but it is a simple fact that our foods are filled with them, and we can't be certain that all of them are fine for us. It may not be possible for us to get rid of these chemicals in our lives completely, but we can get rid of the ones that do end up in our bodies using the natural cleansing process of autophagy.

Not only will you get rid of these toxins for the sake of your general health, but having a clean system leaves you feeling great, too. You can really feel the difference subjectively. We talk so much about the physical health side of things in this book, but we can't ignore the emotional element. Having the peace of mind that your body is consistently getting rid of toxins can be relieving in trying times. Using intermittent fasting is not only about optimizing your physical health as much as possible, but your psychological health as well.

When the detox is a big part of what you want autophagy to do for you, you may be motivated to make it as potent as possible by using a variety of autophagy-triggering methods. Intermittent fasting should be your main method of triggering autophagy since it is the easiest, and therefore, the most reliable. But once you start feeling the difference in your skin and under it — once the work your cells are doing is a sensation you detect throughout your biological systems — there is a good chance you will fall in love with it and want more.

You can combine intermittent fasting with other techniques to make your detox as powerful as possible. If you have a sauna in your community that you can visit, this is a wonderful place to trigger autophagy. Saunas do so much good for your body, although triggering autophagy is the best. They will make your heart rate go down, improve the circulation of your blood, and do a detox on your body directly through your skin. Saunas do this because they put your cells into a state of stress. If you recall, this state of stress is the thing that puts your cells into autophagy. Intermittent fasting is the best way to trigger the state of stress on a daily, reliable basis, but saunas will help, too, giving you the best natural detox possible.

Even if you don't have a sauna, you can get some of the benefits of taking a hot shower. The steam will seep into your skin and do some of the detoxification that a sauna would do. Your cells will get some of the state of stress that would come from a sauna. None of this is to say that a sauna or hot shower should replace intermittent fasting — they shouldn't, because they don't advance autophagy as much as fasting. However, if you use these methods alongside intermittent fasting, the autophagy you get will increase.

Autophagy and Your Skin

Now that you know more about the science of autophagy, we can go deeper into the health benefits that intermittent fasting will confer to your skin.

First of all, you should know how important hydration is to your skin. You may be going through autophagy 12 hours a day and still not see improvement in your skin. Most people do not get enough water every day. Be sure you are drinking 7 glasses a day, at the very least. This is truthfully the best thing you can do for your skin.

Earlier, you learned how intermittent fasting and autophagy detoxify your system. Well, this means that your pores are cleared out, too. No one wants to keep their pores clogged, and if you drink plenty of water and keep up your habit of intermittent fasting, you won't have to worry about clogged pores in your skin for much longer.

The way that IF improves your skin works in two ways. For one, it unclogs these pores, since autophagy breaks down the toxins that clog them up. But IF also makes your skin cells healthier overall. This results in the long-term and more desired effect of more elastic and more youthful skin.

When you keep your skin healthy with autophagy, your true goal is to increase the amount of collagen that your skin cells produce. We went into this topic in the last chapter, but now we have the space to go into more detail.

It is actually not all of your skin cells that produce the collagen protein, but just some of them. These skin cells are called fibroblasts. Fibroblasts are specialized cells made to produce the protein we have been talking about known as collagen.

You can't go wrong with collagen — the more you have of it, the healthier and more elastic your skin is. Even when we turn 18, our fibroblasts start producing less collagen, and our skin starts getting less stretchy as a result. If you want more collagen, you have to take care of your cells by drinking lots of water and doing IF to trigger autophagy. Our fibroblasts stop making as much collagen because they get clogged up with toxins, just like our pores. These cells are not as efficient since they are so crowded out by toxins. The unused proteins, organelles, and other toxins start to add up and create real problems for your fibroblast's functioning.

This is what we mean when we say that autophagy helps your skin in two ways. Because IF triggers autophagy to clean out your pores, but this reduction in toxins also ends up making your fibroblasts healthier and more efficient. More efficient cells are able to do their job properly; fibroblasts get better at producing collagen, and your skin gets tighter.

Taking care of your skin is not only a matter of appearance, although there is nothing wrong with wanting to manage your looks too. Your skin is one of your most important organs. Healthier skin protects you against skin cancer, ultraviolet rays, and diseases trying to permeate through your skin cells' membranes.

The cells of your skin organ are a great example of autophagy in general because skin cells get replaced a lot — all of them get replaced every month. Autophagy is integral to this non-stop process of renewal in your skin cells. Triggering it with IF will result in these health benefits because you are protecting the continuous cycle of skin cells that you need to protect your body.

When you want to detoxify your body, your skin is the best place to do it. It serves as your first line of defense against the toxins that enter your body from the outside.

Autophagy is the best way to get better, healthier skin because it has the capacity to tackle this continual cycle of new cells in your skin. No other method can deal with the constant stream of new skin cells, which is why they tend to fail.

For instance, there are endless skincare products that claim to do what autophagy really does for your skin, but this is impossible since these products can't compete with the way autophagy goes deep into your layers of skin, to your old cells and new cells.

These skincare products can only put creme on top of your outermost layer of skin, making it look better. But it is only covering it up without solving the problem that can only be solved through cellular means.

It is unfortunate that so many people waste their time and money on products that don't work, but at least you won't have to. In fact, the improved health and youthfulness of your skin will probably be the first thing you notice as a result of intermittent fasting. Along with weight loss, it is commonly reported as the first noticeable difference.

The desire to lose weight and get better skin often go together. One reason for this is fear of the so-called "skin curtain." We already discussed this fear briefly, but I want to be sure that you do not let this irrational fear hold you back from making lifestyle changes that are good for your body and your autophagy. Like we said before, loose skin from weight loss has a lot of factors that go into it: (1) the speed at which you lose the weight, (2) how much weight is lost, (3) genetics, (4) age, and (5) the health of your skin. Not only can we deal with loose skin to once you have it, a lot of these things can be prevented in the first place. We can control them. Let's get into controlling loose skin once we have it, though.

Probably the biggest reason we shouldn't worry about loose skin from weight loss is that it isn't permanent. Of course, these things always go on a case-by-case basis, but most people who are looking at loose skin after weight loss don't have to accept it into their lives. There are a variety of ways that it can be managed once you have it, and surgery isn't the only option. Working to get rid of loose skin is a lot like taking care of your skin in general. You want to drive 7 or more glasses of water a day, be getting exercise, get the essential nutrients you should be getting anyway, and do intermittent fasting to stimulate autophagy.

It takes time to tighten up your loose skin, for sure, but this is a much easier problem to deal with than excess fat on your body. It is amazing how many people are reluctant to lose weight because of their irrational fear of loose skin; don't let yourself be one of them. In short, loose skin can be handled once you lose the weight. It is not permanent, just like being overweight or obese isn't permanent. Just like those things, you just have to put in the work consistently and be patient as time does its part in tightening up loose skin from weight loss.

You can keep the loose skin from being a problem in the first place, too. Your age and how much weight you need to lose are not things that you can control, but you can control other things: how much water you drink, how quickly you lose the weight, whether you get enough nutrients, and whether you exercise.

Most importantly, you can do intermittent fasting to trigger autophagy, and this will help with loose skin the most. It has been shown in research that people who fast deal with less loose skin when they lose the weight they want to lose. Take care of the things you can control, and if you still have some loose skin when the weight is off, keep taking care of your body and following your IF routine so your skin tightens as quickly as possible.

You can pay attention to how you feel when you fast to help prevent loose skin in the first place. Many people say that when they do a longer fast like a water fast that their skin feels strange. You can feel this slightly without worrying about it, but if the feeling goes further than that, you might want to stop your fast early. It could be that your skin is not adjusting to your new body shape quickly enough, and if the fast continues, you will have the loose skin that you don't want.

It's true that your skin is the organ that everyone can see, and this is why there is a multi-million-dollar industry to helping people improve their skin health. However, the way your skin looks should not be the main thing that you are concerned about. It is just like how people want to lose weight to look better but losing weight will also decrease their health risks for heart disease and cancer, too. Women, in particular, need to pay close attention to the health of their skin, because sometimes they use so many products on them that they are unsure of the natural state of their skin health.

After you take a shower, inspect your skin and evaluate how healthy you think it is. Inspecting your skin regularly will get you motivated to keep on your IF regimen. You will see improvements very quickly. Your skin's purpose is not to look nice, but to protect your body from toxins on the outside. Doing IF will help you protect your skin, empowering it to shield your system from pathogens and microbes. Thankfully, taking care of your skin will also make it look better. It is a win-win situation.

Autophagy and Your Energy

Everyone who fasts says the same thing: they can do so much more now every day than they used to be able to because they have more energy.

You already know that everything that you do requires energy — and this is true all the way down to your cells. Your cells, in a sense, need more energy than you do, because they have to keep doing their jobs 24/7. They will break down organelles and proteins that no longer help them when you deprive them of food because they always need to find energy somewhere.

If you don't trigger autophagy except when you are sleeping, a lot of negative consequences are likely — one of them being low energy. Many people who don't have much energy feel this way because their cells are not running optimally. Their cells are having to drag along all their cellular waste getting in the way. If you don't fast to force them to clean this out, they will still do it, but not nearly enough.

The mitochondria are where all of your energy starts. This is the organelle where your cell makes energy so it can perform all the jobs that it has to do. This chapter focuses on the benefits that IF and autophagy have for your body, but it is useful to think about things from a microscopic point of view, too. The mitochondrion is arguably the most important organelle in your cells. If your mitochondrion is working well, this is a sign that your cell is working well. When scientists look at mitochondrial health in people, they find that those with well-functioning mitochondria are at low risk for neurodegenerative diseases like Huntington's, Alzheimer's, and Parkinson's.

Your mitochondria do their job best when they don't have to deal with clutter. Clutter builds up around your mitochondria in their cell from all the sources we have mentioned, and this slows it down. When you don't trigger autophagy enough, this has consequences for mitochondria all over your body — consequences for the one place where all your energy ultimately comes from. It's no wonder that people who fast have more energy.

Their cells' power plants are working better than they ever have before!

It is likely that you have heard of ATP before. ATP is the particle that is fundamental to your body's energy at an atomic level. ATP is where all of your cells get their energy. It doesn't matter whether your cells get energy from breaking down your food or from breaking down toxins — ATP is at the center of the process.

The details of ATP breakdown are truly fascinating, but for our purposes, we can summarize by saying that your cells use the energy that comes from converting ATP into ADP and back into ATP again (and so on).Now, this process of ATP breakdown doesn't require energy because it's how we get energy. But it does require two things: oxygen and nourishment. All living things break down ATP, be they animals or plants. The main difference is animals use oxidation, and plants use photosynthesis.

The fascinating truth about ATP is that your system generates around 170 pounds of it each day, despite the fact that there are only around 9 ounces of ATP in your body at any given time. You only ever have half a pound of ATP in your body, yet the process of transformation of ATP, giving your body energy goes through the weight of a human. The process of ATP breakdown occurs in the mitochondria of all of your cells. When you let ATP happen using toxins, dead organelles, and proteins during intermittent fasting, this makes the process much more effective.

Remember: your cells don't have brains like you do, because if they did, they would know that they should clean themselves out to make ATP breakdown happen more smoothly. But now that you know this yourself, this is no longer a problem. Make intermittent fasting a regular part of your life and start seeing your energy levels spike.

Autophagy: It's What's Good for You

The fact is, not everyone thinks as much about their general health as they should. The sad thing is that once you are diagnosed with something that could have been prevented, you wish that you had thought more about taking care of your body.

If you are reading now and you aren't currently looking at a major health crisis, the good thing is that it isn't too late yet. You can still turn around your attitude of health and start caring about it. We are primarily focused on what autophagy can do for your health through intermittent fasting, but the habits that make autophagy more potent are the same ones that you should keep up for the betterment of your health in general.

It should be enough to tell you that intermittent fasting reduces your risk for neurodegenerative diseases. The older you get, the higher your chances of getting one of these becomes. It is within your power to lower your risk, and these new habits don't just increase the length of your life. They make you feel better too, improving the quality of your life.

We won't spend too much more time on Alzheimer's and the rest since we have already talked about them a lot. But diabetes is a disease that should not be taken lightly, either. Many people live with diabetes, but that doesn't mean it has no consequences. If you don't have it already, it is certainly worth the change in lifestyle to avoid it.

IF is a great path to staying away from diabetes. People who get this disease end up with amyloid deposits in their arteries, but if their cells had broken down the amyloid during autophagy, they wouldn't have gotten diabetes in the first place. Scientists are still learning more about the potential of autophagy to treat these diseases, but what we can already do is stop them in their tracks through fasting.

You can look at the positive effects of autophagy on your overall health from two different angles. First and most obviously, there is the angle of stopping microbes and pathogens before they become an issue. If your body is in the mode of autophagy half the time because you are passionate about autophagy and fasting, there is a very good chance you will rarely have to worry about infection — because your cells always deal with them very early.

This is the purpose of advanced autophagy. You will go through what biologists call "maintenance mode" autophagy no matter what your body habits are. No one in the world eats every moment of the day, and everyone has to sleep. During these periods of time, our cells still need energy, so they have to go through autophagy to get food with which to go through ATP breakdown.

Intermittent fasting spurs the biological process that puts a stopper on many risks for age-related disease: high inflammation, high blood pressure, being overweight, and more. Autophagy's lowering of inflammation is often underappreciated in research. Inflammation is something that can speed up the progression of disease when something else is wrong. You may have an infection, but if you have a relatively low level of inflammation, there is a good chance that your body will eventually take care of it. If you have high inflammation and you get an infection, however, the issue is compounded. Your system is sluggish and doesn't fight off the pathogen before it is too late.

The earlier you start IF, the better, because your autophagy won't be as potent at first. Even if you do everything right — paying attention to your nutrients, not consuming too many calories, exercising, drinking enough water, and following your IF regimen — your first month or so of fasting won't do nearly as much as the months after. It takes time for your body to break toxins down. If you had not ever fasted before, your autophagy is now working on a backlog of old toxins that will take time to get there. Luckily, once this is finished, your autophagy will be better than ever.

And on the subject of inflammation, once autophagy decreases your inflammation, autophagy will be more effective as well. If you have not talked to your doctor about inflammation before, you might not be sure if yours is high or not. You might have high inflammation if you have bad habits like smoking, overeating, alcohol abuse, or following a sedentary lifestyle.

Some of the most recent studies about autophagy have shown that a low amount of it is the cause of neurodegenerative diseases. I may have already made clear that autophagy fights against these diseases, but now you should know precisely why. It all has to do with a special kind of autophagy: chaperone-mediated autophagy. We will go into more detail on what this distinction means later one. This is what you need to know for now, though — biologists found that the gene instructing your cells to go through chaperone-mediated autophagy was damaged in people with neurodegenerative diseases. Since the gene was damaged, they did not go through chaperone-mediated autophagy when they should have. Next, proteins piled up inside the brain cells of people with these diseases. The buildup of protein gets to a point where the brain cells don't work properly anymore, and they die.

There is another theory on how it happens, but it has the same result. Other scientists think that the autophagosome (transporter essential to chaperone-mediated autophagy and macroautophagy) binds to the lysosome (cell stomach) too strongly. As a result, there is a clogging effect, and too many proteins crowded into a cell, leading to its dysfunction and eventual death. It can be tempting to think that such things are inevitable. It can seem like you can't do anything about what happens in your brain cells. You think, just let it be. It is outside of my control. But this is not true at all. There are many people who do not ever get these diseases. Of course, we cannot deny that genes play a role, but saying that genes determine everything is just a way of not doing what we can.

Let's assume that the scientists who say neurodegeneration happens because of the "clogging effect" are right. The way you should look at it is that you can still prevent the issue from getting out of hand, just like you can with infections. When the clogging effect happens in people's brain cells, it doesn't happen in every single one.

This gives you the opportunity to trigger autophagy in the cells without the clogging effect so they can clean out the protein buildups before they get out of hand. If you do this on a regular basis, you won't have to have the stress of a damaged gene.

Your cells inevitably age just like we do and get damaged genes. This doesn't mean that we should give up on them and simply allow them to not work as well as they could. Our cells without damaged DNA can pick up the slack for the ones who do. Besides, chaperone-mediated autophagy has another role that we have not yet gotten to. Scientists were excited to see that this special kind of autophagy is actually responsible for repairing your cells' DNA.

If you use IF regularly — especially if you are making autophagy unleash to its fullest extent — you can even repair the genes that prevent autophagy from working the way it should. IF and autophagy can teach all of us to take more initiative with our health. When you learn how much control we really have, it can serve as quite a wake-up call. All you need is the knowledge of how it works and the will to live healthily for as long as possible.

Chapter 4:
Intermittent Fasting and Autophagy

At the heart of intermittent fasting's benefits is the science that makes all of it work. Autophagy is the biological process in which your cells, when unable to get energy from food, consume "junk" materials such as unused organelles, proteins, and foreign toxins.

You put your body through autophagy when you do intermittent fasting because you are depriving your cells of food to consume, so they switch to autophagy to get their energy. Because of this, you can reap all the advantages of autophagy by simply not eating during certain windows of the day.

This will be the chapter where we dive into the biological component of intermittent fasting, the process that we aim to achieve by fasting autophagy. I know that science is not everyone's cup of tea, but you need to know this essential information, so you know how to best set up your IF routine.

Even if you are a fan of learning about science, it is easy to get overwhelmed with information overload, especially when you only learned about autophagy recently. But there are some simple facts that will make things easier for you. Firstly, I am not leaving out anything important in this chapter. You can rest easy knowing that you are not missing something important about autophagy in this chapter.

The other simple fact is that I am still only telling you what you need to know. Put together, what I'm saying is that you don't need to check other sources to learn the science of autophagy, because this one is exhaustive, and you don't need to worry about reading more information than you can absorb, because I am telling you what you need to know and nothing more. This science-based chapter is woven in such a way that you do not have to worry about accidentally skipping something important. Everything is connected and related to each other. All you have to do is continue reading the chapter from start to finish, and your job is done.

Part of the reason learning the science behind intermittent fasting is so important is because you need to be certain of autophagy's significance yourself. If you can't tell your friends in a few sentences why you are doing intermittent fasting, you will lose sight of the purpose of it, and you might be in danger of stopping. You will have more than a few sentences to say to back up the science of intermittent fasting after reading this chapter. It is probable that you might annoy your friends with facts about autophagy for a week or so after reading.

They might be annoyed with you, but they won't be able to discredit the points your making, so you will probably be doing their health a favor. Doing intermittent fasting is a lot more fun when you have friends or family doing it with you, so learning the ins and outs of the science behind intermittent fasting is a great opportunity to recruit others to help you live more healthily.

Where It All Started

There is a history that accompanies the study of autophagy and all the things we know about it regarding our health. Autophagy was a term that people might use for its philosophical meaning that can be gleaned from "self" "eat" (autophagy), but even using the term to refer to a specific biological phenomenon is a new thing.

The first scientist to get close to learning about autophagy is Christian De Duve, and he was the first one to use the term autophagy. However, his understanding of it is so different from what we think of it now, that it is almost like he was studying something else entirely. In France in the 1960's, Christian De Duve saw a new organelle while looking at yeast cells in the laboratory. Since it had never been identified before, his team of researchers started learning all the bizarre things about it. They called this organelle the "lysosome." The lysosome was understood quite differently back then, though. Christian De Duve still called the lysosome the center of autophagy because he concluded that this was the garbage receptacle of the cell.

You can see how scientists got some things right, but most things wrong. It makes sense, given that they had only just discovered the site of autophagy, but biological understanding has gone far past seeing the lysosome and autophagy this way.

It was very recently that our understanding evolved to what it is today. The Japanese scientists Yoshinori Ohsumi won the Nobel Prize for re-defining autophagy into how we see it today. Ohsumi studied yeast cells too, but unlike Christian De Duve, yeast cells were the basis of his entire career. To this day, his team is still trying to learn more about autophagy, and they are still using yeast cells to do this. From reading so far, you already know what Ohsumi learned from looking at the lysosomes of yeast cells. We now know that autophagy is not simply a process of disposal, but a process of recycling.

This makes a lot more sense, too, because there is no such thing as "breaking something down" in the real world so it turns into nothing. We can only change the form of matter; we can't actually destroy it. Ohsumi incorporated the "recycling" aspect of autophagy by being the first to talk about what he calls the "cell cycle." The cell cycle is the means by which your cells break down their toxins in the lysosome and then use the raw materials left behind to build new things. With the raw materials collected from autophagy, our cells can build new organelles and new cells.

The cell cycle is how our cells use their waste to create cellular structures, and then those structures break down their waste to create their own structures, and so forth. It is interesting that we did not think of our cells this way until the last few years, because in retrospect, we know that it is one of the essential jobs that your cells must do.

Ohsumi's research has gotten pharmacists started on medicines that can use our knowledge of autophagy to fight aging and age-related disease. They could find something revolutionary that could change medicine forever any day. In the meantime, we can make the best use out of what we already know.

Now that you know the context under which autophagy has been studied — and now that you know how cutting-edge autophagy really is — we will explore the different kinds of autophagy that exist and how they apply to intermittent fasting.

Microautophagy

This is the form that autophagy takes in every single cell of your body. All cells have lysosomes, and those lysosomes have the chief purpose of conducting microautophagy. As usual, their job is to bring in damaged organelles to break them down. This is different from macroautophagy and chaperone-mediated autophagy, where the lysosome does not pull in the cellular waste on its own. In those kinds of autophagy, a special organelle called the autophagosome has the job of finding waste inside and outside of the cell. Then, it carries them over to the lysosome and binds with it to break down its contents.

Microautophagy happens in every cell because it does some very important jobs. It helps with the homeostasis of the membrane and it keeps the cell's organelles at their current size.

The chemical function of the lysosome is still being studied, but essentially its method of breaking down the cellular waste is attacking them with enzymes. Finally, microautophagy is finished and the cell uses the raw materials attained from breaking down the waste for its part of the cell cycle. The cell can use the materials for building a new cell, building a new organelle, or for building even more basic things like glucose, amino acids, fatty acids, and so forth.

Macroautophagy

Macroautophagy is the type of autophagy that is only seen in cells with certain jobs. This type and chaperone-mediated autophagy use the autophagosome. The autophagosome can be simply described as a vesicle — that is, it can carry things inside of it and transport them. This vesicle (the autophagosome) travels around inside the cell and goes outside the cell to find waste to break down when you are fasting, and food is scarce. When it is done wandering through the cytoplasm finding waste, it returns to the lysosome and binds with it.

When the autophagosome takes the materials into the lysosome, this is called sequestration. The autophagosome has a double membrane around it that it uses to trap materials inside. When sequestration occurs, both membranes open so that the lysosome can take the toxins that the vesicle found. But in macroautophagy, it is not the lysosome that breaks down the toxins, but the autophagosome. It can only break them down when it is bonded to the lysosome, however.

Since macroautophagy only happens in specialized cells like white blood cells, there are actually a few different kinds of macroautophagy itself, such as mitophagy and ribophagy. Most of the time, these different kinds of macroautophagy are made for getting rid of specific organelles that have stopped working.

Chaperone-Mediated Autophagy

The direction of biology and medicine may hinge on our newest findings about this kind of autophagy: chaperone-mediated autophagy. Scientists have known about the other two types of autophagy for much longer than chaperone-mediated autophagy; it was Yoshinori Ohsumi's research that led to the interest in autophagy that spurred its discovery. The findings that we have so far will influence science and medicine for decades to come.

Chaperone-mediated autophagy is the most specialized kind of autophagy of the three. Essentially, this kind of autophagy differentiates itself because it uses chains of proteins to move materials into the lysosome. The proteins themselves are specialized for this one purpose in chaperone-mediated autophagy, and the materials they help move into the lysosome are specific proteins that CMA seeks after.

In our chapter about the benefits of autophagy, we went into CMA briefly because of its job of DNA repair. I am about to go into all the wonders of chaperone-mediated autophagy and what we know about it so far, but we can summarize the most important facts about CMA briefly.

For one, chaperone-mediated autophagy does not only break down proteins. It has a vital role in repairing DNA. As we learned earlier, the DNA repair of cells is very important, because damaged DNA leads to cells not performing as they should be. When your brain cells have damaged genes, they don't perform autophagy when they should, and the result is buildups of proteins that lead to Alzheimer's, Parkinson's, and Huntington's.

Next, CMA is important because it seeks after specific proteins to break them down. This is crucial because if CMA did not do this, the raw materials from those proteins could be lacking in a cell and it wouldn't be able to proceed in the cell cycle as efficiently.

Besides these two important jobs, chaperone-mediated autophagy has some others, too. Studies have concluded that CMA plays a role in your cell metabolism and in controlling your glucose levels. Keeping your glucose relatively low is what makes autophagy possible in the first place.

Microautophagy and macroautophagy might end up breaking down important proteins for the raw materials they need, but they can't use specialized protein chains to seek specific proteins out.

Cells that perform CMA know which proteins to seek out because of the instructions from their genes. It is useful that CMA is also needed to repair the DNA of cells, because it needs that DNA to do its job.

In the last chapter, we learned that the precursor to Alzheimer's and similar diseases is damaged DNA inside cells. I told you that you shouldn't accept this as something you can't control, because using autophagy, you do have the power to fight against damaged DNA and eventual neurodegeneration.

You can use this book as a life-changing resource to optimize the effects of autophagy and repair your cell DNA as often as possible. Anything you could ever need to know about how to do this is contained in here.

While we are getting more in the weeds about chaperone-mediated autophagy, you should learn about the latest gene related to it: LAMP-2A. This name stands for lysosome-associated membrane protein.

We know a few things about this gene already: (1) it has a strong link to chaperone-mediated autophagy and (2) when scientists preserve this gene in lab mice, they had better outcomes in health and longer lifespans than mice without having this gene protected. One scientist even noted that the mice whose LAMP-2A was protected had "healthier-looking fur" and "a glow about them."

If these symptoms sound familiar, it's because they are close to the ones that humans experience when they trigger autophagy by fasting. Your skin gets a glow, and while we don't have fur, there's a good chance the new hair you grow will be healthier, too.

When I told you that chaperone-mediated autophagy could repair DNA, regulate metabolism, and control glucose levels, all of these jobs are actually due to instructions that your cells get from their LAMP-2A gene. It's also the gene that probably gets damaged in people who develop neurodegenerative diseases.

The LAMP-2A gene is supposed to tell your specialized cells to start chaperone-mediated autophagy and seek out the specific proteins named in their DNA. When these

96

genes are damaged, your autophagy does not function as it is supposed to, and all the biological processes that rely on it start to have problems as well.

Some of the recent findings about autophagy have turned out to be incredibly relevant to matters of personal health. It has only been in the past decade that we found out that Alzheimer's and Parkinson's disease are a result of a mutation in a gene that controls autophagy.

Let's step back for a second and define what we mean by mutation. As we age, the DNA in our cells becomes damaged from wear and tear. One of the genes in our DNA is the one that controls autophagy. When that gene takes damage, our autophagy is less effective because it is not getting proper instructions from the DNA.

As a result, when your brain cells create protein chains to do certain jobs, these protein chains become clusters that are toxic to your cells, all because these cells did not have undamaged genes from which to take their instructions.

Now you might worry that this gene damage as a result of age means that there is nothing you can do about it, but this could not be further from the truth. Your takeaway from this scientific discovery should be that you need to manually turn on autophagy as you get older because your cells' genes will not be as effective at doing it automatically. You can turn on autophagy through fasting and exercise and get the same much-needed autophagy as you would if your genes instructed your cells to do it to themselves.

Microscopic is Everything

Perhaps you are a reader who is skeptical about something so small having such an impact. You believe that all the science is true, but you don't think that your cells are what you should focus on, when you could focus on your specific organs or certain muscles.

It might help for you to think of yourself as one big cell. As you, the cell, age, you take damage. Cells that have gone through damage do not work as well until they go through autophagy and fix their injuries.

In much the same way, you as a person can suffer injuries, and those injuries impede your ability to do what you need to do. If you got in an accident tomorrow and broke your hand, there are a lot of things you wouldn't be able to do. Even if you don't have to go to work, things that used to be simple — like getting the mail — are not simple anymore.

A cell with an injury to the mitochondria is not in the right state to cooperate with the rest of your cells. Ultimately, we are talking about just one cell here, and it doesn't do any good alone — especially if it is injured and not working properly.

It might seem like one cell doesn't matter, but you have over 30 trillion cells in your whole body. That's 30,000,000,000,000 cells.

You aren't made of anything else, either. Just cells. Even though one cell admittedly doesn't matter, issues arise when cells throughout your body aren't getting enough autophagy.

There is even a process of programmed cell death that your cell might run if they are too damaged to help the rest of the tissue. They also might do this if they are starting to become a cancer cell; that way, they do not hurt the rest of the body.

Since autophagy disposes of cellular waste and builds new cell structures throughout all of your cells, it is your best defense against threats to your health: and autophagy happens in your microscopic cells. There is no real way to talk about your autophagy outside of your cells, at least when it comes to biology.

You can't do a single thing you do without your cells, so don't underestimate them. Don't underestimate the harmful effects of DNA damage in your cells and the buildup of toxins inside them.

When we age, our cells get less effective. They are less effective because their organelles are less effective. When you have a mitochondrion or another organelle that does not perform well, it is really better to break it down and make it a new mitochondrion. Getting your cells to do this will result in better overall health for you.

However, your cells don't know this like you do. If you want them to get rid of the bad orangeades that are making them lag behind, you have to trigger autophagy by yourself. You have already learned some of the methods that people can use to do this: intermittent fasting, water fasting, a nutrient-rich diet, exercise, a hot shower, or even a sauna will do the trick.

Your cells might not take care of their poorly performing organelles if you do not use these techniques. They might continue using the same old mitochondria without even improving it. When a lot of your cells do this, you end up feeling a difference subjectively.

The health of your cells is the health of your body. You can't micromanage trillions of cells, but you can be a puppet master and manipulate them to do what you want as best as you can.

Take a broken-down vehicle as an example. You might feel emotionally attached to a car that stopped working, but that doesn't mean that you should hold onto it forever. For the first few times that it broke down, you bought the new parts and simply fixed the car. It didn't work as well as before, and it made some suspicious noises, but you like the car, so you allowed it.

But then there is the final straw. You have put thousands of dollars into the car, and at this point, even though you have an attachment to it, you can't justify spending all this money on a car that will just keep breaking down soon after you fix it.

You might say that your cells get attached to their organelles. They don't literally, of course, but they certainly won't get rid of them until they absolutely have to.

This illustrates your cells working in maintenance mode. When you use all of the methods to trigger advanced autophagy together, you can basically communicate with your cells, saying: "I want you to take out the trash."

Your cells need the energy, and they will dig into their reserves. If you spent many years without fasting and without following a generally healthy lifestyle, there is a good chance that it will take time for your cells to break down their problematic organelles. That's because they have so many other options for energy that have stacked up over the years.

After you do intermittent fasting for enough time, though, your cells will finally run out of options and break down their mitochondria. Then, they will use the parts to build a new one. You will surely feel a difference after just a week or so doing intermittent fasting, but this is why the biggest difference in energy levels will be after a longer period of time.

You have likely heard before that humans can live for three weeks or so without eating anything. Autophagy is the reason this is true. At the end of the day, it isn't "you" who has to eat, but your cells. Your cells keep your body alive for weeks because there is plenty already inside of you that they can consume for energy.

But it isn't only when you are starving that your cells break down this much material. Did you know that we need around 100 grams of protein each day? It sounds like a lot, but the reason the number is so high is that you actually only get about one-third of this protein from the foods that you consume.

The only two-thirds of the proteins that your body breaks down every day are protein already inside you. This is autophagy. Even before you knew what it was, it was supplying twice the volume of protein than you were consuming yourself. In other words, your cells don't just break down the protein you eat once. They break it down several times until it is eventually converted into a useful structure. Then that cellular structure stops functioning in the required way, autophagy breaks it down, and it continues on and on.

Another strange thing about this microscopic phenomenon is that you don't have to do anything special to get your body to do it. It is doing it right now, and it will continue to do it for as long as you live. You didn't do anything special to harm your proteins and organelles, either — they simply accrued damage over time while you were going about your normal life.

Autophagy is an essential biological process that will continue whether you decide to pay attention to it or not. But think about this: why would you not want to pay close attention to a process this important? A process that has been instrumental in keeping you alive to this point?

You have the option to add to the power of autophagy by changing your way of living: your eating habits and your exercise habits. We all know that the older we get, the more work we have to do to make our bodies perform the way that they should. But usually, we hear this about our organs, our bones, and our muscles. For some reason, no one says this about autophagy — even though none of these systems would function without it.

The Newest Science

It can be exciting to learn about new scientific discoveries, and the newer the discoveries are, the more exciting they are. This is our final section in the chapter about the science underlying intermittent fasting, and it will concentrate on the newest information that we have about autophagy.

Just keep in mind that these findings are the definition of cutting-edge, meaning there is probably more information about them by the time you read this. You might want to do some research for yourself to see if anything new has been discovered. With that said, at the time of writing, these are the latest findings we have.

To begin, there is another important gene in autophagy besides the LAMP-2A gene. It is called ATG. ATG doesn't stand for anything — it's just supposed to look like the word "autophagy" since its main purpose is to instruct autophagy.

The ATG gene is often discussed alongside the protein chain VPS-34. Both of them are needed to get autophagy triggered and keep it regulated. While scientists protected the LAMP-2A gene from improving the overall health of mice, they found that they could get the most out of VPS-34 by altering it. The manipulation of this protein chain may be key to treating or even curing age-related diseases.

VPS-34 is an easily manipulated chain, and this makes it a great tool for biologists trying to learn more about autophagy. We know that the beginning of many of the diseases we are talking about is related to the deterioration of functions related to chaperone-mediated autophagy. The ability to manipulate one of the protein chains related to CMA (VPS-34) is a phenomenal step in the right direction for everyone who wants to end diseases like cancer.

Some say that it is only a matter of time before experiments on VPS-34 lead to a new ground-breaking discovery. When that happens, medicine as we know it — especially as it relates to aging — will be totally changed.

There is one more gene you should know: the P62 gene. This gene is often attributed to the relatively long lifespan that humans have compared to other mammals.

It took time for humans to get the P62 gene in our evolution. But what does it do? Maybe you won't be surprised that it is related to chaperone-mediated autophagy: it lets our cells know when there are dangerous products that could harm them, causing them to go into a state of stress and trigger autophagy.

When scientists created genetically mutated fruit flies and gave them the P62 gene, they survived for longer than fruit flies without the P62 gene. This experiment alone should convince you of the singular potential of autophagy.

Now that you have a strong grasp on the research for cancer and neurodegenerative diseases, we should spend some time on another important disease: diabetes. Then, I will recommend what foods to eat when you are following a routine of intermittent fasting in the next chapter.

You might remember learning about amyloid deposits, the buildups of proteins that lead to diabetes. There is a lesson to be learned in all these cases of diseases that could be prevented with more autophagy; they are not caused by a foreign invader. They are caused by our bodies working seemingly normally — until an invisible line is crossed, and too much protein accumulates in the cells.

If there is only one takeaway you have from this science-focused chapter, it should be that increased autophagy prevents the diseases that we can't otherwise address until it's too late.

You can't tell when your proteins are crowded out your brain cells or cells anywhere else; the only way you can prevent it from becoming a problem is by fasting regularly. If you do that, you will know that you are doing everything you can do to stave off diseases for which there is no other real treatment.

Chapter 5:
Food to Eat During
Intermittent Fasting

If there is one thing to remember in an intermittent fast, it's this: lower your consumption of carbohydrates. The reason for this is that carbs take a long time for your body to process, and as long as your body is processing food, it is not starting autophagy yet.

This ends up reducing the amount of time your body goes through autophagy. Carbs are also the first thing your gut decides to break down — it will break down carbs before protein or fat. With that important tip in mind, let's get into the best foods to eat if you want to maximize the good your body gets from intermittent fasting.

Your general guiding principle needs to be that you have to stop eating without thinking — that is, you need to recognize the different physical and mental consequences that you will have because of the foods that you eat. Once you get really good at following this principle, all the other tips that you hear just seem like common sense.

To quickly review the foods we previously told you help with autophagy, they are the reishi mushroom, turmeric, green tea, caffeine, olive oil, and ginger.

All of these foods contain chemicals that will help your body have better autophagy when you trigger it, but they will not trigger autophagy alone — not without fasting or exercise. Don't get that mixed up.

There are still more foods that you might consider. Grapes have also been found to help with autophagy, for example. CBD, the non-psychoactive brother of THC, is proved to help autophagy as well. CBD works particularly well for this purpose because it lessens the amount of inflammation in your body while also improving your neural connections leading the charge with autophagy.

You don't want to spend too much time thinking about what special foods to eat — at least not until you get to a point with IF where you can trust yourself to do it without slipping. When that happens, it can be an exciting way to mix things up.

Ultimately, eating these foods is just doing extra to make your autophagy more advanced. More important than eating these specific foods is getting a balanced diet when you are not inside your fasting window. The rest of the chapter will focus on this because it is much more important.

The best diet for intermittent fasting isn't just the best diet for intermittent fasting because it is a diet filled with the foods that you should be getting, whether you fast or not.

To get the full potential of autophagy while you do IF, you are best off following this plan, but it does not have to constrain you absolutely. As we said before, the choices you make with your body are yours to make. Even saying that, though, there are certain foods you want to make sure not to eat because they will interfere with your autophagy badly.

I won't make too fine a point on carbs, because you get the message at this point. There is just one other thing to add, which is that even if you fall out of fasting sometime in the future, you still want to greatly reduce the proportion of it in your diet.

They say that Americans are overweight because of sugar and fats, and this is partly true, but the true culprit is carbohydrates. Carbs are the "fluff" of nutrients — they take up a lot of space compared to others, and it is very easy to get too much of it.

Do not misinterpret this and think that you should stay away from carbs altogether. You need carbs just like you need all of these foods. However, it is very easy to get the carbs that you need daily without even trying.

Carbs are a lot like protein this way — it isn't hard to figure out where you will get them, most of the time, because they are in a lot of the foods around us.

It is time for you to learn about protein cycling. Protein cycling is a diet change that many people make when they do intermittent fasting. Basically, it means alternating between days of normal protein intake and low protein intake.

It is still important that you eat a normal amount of protein on the normal days because protein is an essential nutrient in your body. You need some level of normal protein every day, so your cells have it to build structures.

However, the low-protein days are important too. Having days where you consume little protein will further spur your cells to turn on autophagy during your fasting window.

Your cells already have plenty of protein lying around as cellular garbage, so your cells can reliably use this as their source of protein on your low-protein days. (Don't forget the fact we learned earlier — your body processes 100 grams of it each day, and only a quarter of that comes from the food you eat!)

With all that in mind, you never want to consume lots of protein, no matter how important a nutrient it is. There is a very good reason for this. When you eat lots of protein, all you are doing is giving your cells lots of cellular garbage to clean out during autophagy.

Your cells have to cycle between normal, non-stressed periods and autophagy periods, so it takes time for your cells to get rid of all of this excess.

When they take too long to do it, it eventually becomes toxic, as we have learned. Despite how essential a nutrient protein is, there is such thing as too much of a good thing, especially when it comes to protein.

When your diet is very high in protein, this hampers the progress of autophagy greatly. It does not hamper its progress as much as carbohydrates do, but it still slows things down. Instead of cleaning out your existing cellular garbage when you do IF, you will simply be cleaning out the junk left behind by all the protein you just ate.

Protein cycling gives us a great chance to discuss the importance of finding a balance between IF and a healthy diet. When you do protein cycling, you still need to eat the recommended amount of protein for a reason: it is an essential nutrient.

However, you can go too far in either direction. A lot of the foods people love contain protein, so it is common for people to eat far more protein than they should without even realizing it.

On the other hand, starving yourself of protein to the extreme is harmful, too. If you do this, you may experience loss in muscle tone that is usually associated with fasts more extreme than intermittent fasting.

To do protein cycling right, simply eat the recommended amount of protein every other day, and half or less that amount on your other days.

This is not only about protein, though. Even though IF is a fast meant for everyone, there are still ways we can take it too far. Take someone who makes their fasting window too long: let's say, 14 hours. That would mean they eat for an hour in the morning and then eat again for an hour before bed. This is absolutely unhealthy, and I strongly recommend avoiding it.

I especially advise against it because the IF is meant to be done every day. If you are fasting for 14 hours every day, that could have serious consequences on your body. With a water fast, you may fast for as much as 24 or 48 hours, but the difference is the frequency. Someone can do a water fast all day on Sunday and then go back to their normal eating patterns on Monday.

But if they do IF for 14 hours a day, there is never a time they return to their regular eating pattern. Their regular eating pattern involves consuming far too infrequently.

Maybe you are familiar with the concept of yin and yang from Taoism. The yang gives, and the yin takes. To find a balance between a healthy diet and IF, keep thinking of eating as yang and IF as yin. You need yang to fill yourself up with fresh nutrients.

When you are following IF, you do this outside of your fasting window. You need yin to cleanse your cells of the toxins produced from yang.

Too much of yang (eating) and too much of yin (fasting) both have negative consequences. The key is to find a balance between the two; this will allow you to get the benefits of both.

Put another way, don't let yourself believe that "extra" fasting will lead to better health outcomes. It won't. If you truly want to be healthy, you need to find the right about eating for your yang and the right amount of fasting for your yin.

There are writers on the subject of water fasting who concede that these drinks will stymie autophagy to some extent, but they say that at the end of the day, it doesn't make much of a difference. I beg to differ. We have a lot of scientific evidence of the effectiveness of pure water fasting — we don't have any evidence to back up a pure water fast, minus some coffee here and there.

Even a cup of coffee at the beginning of your fast can mess things up. Don't take the risk when you are already looking to get as much as possible out of autophagy.

Another common mistake is consuming flavored water during the water fast. Do not do this — again, the flavoring has something that your body has to break down. When your body breaks down chemicals, autophagy stops. You should even stay away from smells of flavor. It sounds bizarre, but even the smell of real or artificial food causes a parasympathetic reaction from your vagus nerve.

This reaction will actually keep autophagy from happening to a significant degree because it stimulates mTOR, a gene that will stop autophagy when activated. It may feel like there is such a delicate balance, but if you are water fasting to maximize the potential of autophagy, these are the things you have to consider.

Don't even take vitamins or supplements that purport to boost autophagy during your water fast. Not to beat a dead horse, but: your body has to process that, and then autophagy won't start until it's done.

People who advocate for these supplements say that supplements don't have enough digestible chemicals to stop autophagy from happening, but they don't really know this is the case. They are just selling a supplement. (On a side note, there is no official supplement that is known to turn on or even aid autophagy at this moment, so you shouldn't bother shopping around for them.)

The list of what to avoid goes on. If it doesn't occur naturally and it comes in colorful packaging, stay away from it. Don't drink soda, eat candy, or buy any of the meat from your grocery store that comes from factory farms. All the nutrients you should be indirectly getting from the grass that animal ate is not there, because these animals are stuffed with chemicals instead of fed grass.

It should probably go without saying, but you need to stay away from sugar as well. Ideally, most of the sugars in your diet come from fruits, and you don't even want to eat too many of those. Even eating more than a little bit of fruit can put too much sugar into your system, so that should tell you how bad sugar is for you.

Sugar may not take as long to digest as carbs, but at least as far as artificial sugars go, you simply don't need it. When you consume too much sugar, you are adding a lot of waste that your cells will have to clean out later with autophagy.

In fact, this is the image that you should conjure with all of the foods you put into your system. Imagine your broken-down, microscopic foods inside your cells. What will be the most useful to your cells (again, your cells make up all of you): sugary foods or foods with tons of vitamins?

We all know the answer, but the harder part is following through. Actually, doing it may not be as hard as you think. Once you have made the decision to do your first intermittent fasting day tomorrow, you should go grocery shopping. This is what makes it easy: all you have to do is refrain from buying the foods that we are talking about.

Don't buy bagels. Don't buy packaged snacks. Don't buy cake mix.

You know what you should buy already. Put dairy products in your cart that have healthy protein. Put in some natural fruit juice and cucumbers. Pick up healthy nuts like cashews. Find a recipe that you think looks tasty and uses the foods that you want to take part of your normal diet.

Recipes are the key to changing your diet. This is for many reasons. Firstly, cooking takes time, and nothing is better than already knowing how to cook something and already having the ingredients. You will also feel good about making food at home, saving money by not going out.

Going out to eat is a big risk, particularly in the early stages of intermittent fasting. I advise you not to go out to eat until you can at least keep yourself from eating during your fast for two weeks.

Now, let's get right to it. What should you be eating when you do the IF?

I know it's not food, but it deserves as much attention, if not more: water. Every system that keeps you alive needs water to keep going, and that doesn't stop being true when you are fasting. The color of your urine will tell you if you are drinking enough water. The clearer it is, the better — although if it is totally clear, that means you are drinking more than enough water.

Another boon of drinking a lot of water during IF is that it keeps your cravings away. A lot of the times we think that we want food, but what we really feel is thirst.

Next, you need to make fish a weekly dish. They are your best source of Omega-3 fats, an important nutrient for autophagy. Fish also have vitamins and protein. The

American Heart Association tells us we should be eating at least one serving of fish every week. Are you?

You may not expect this one, but potatoes are a good food option for IF, too. They are because potatoes are especially filling, while actually giving us real nutrients. Getting full on potatoes will keep you from eating when you are supposed to be fasting. There is even research showing that people with potatoes in their diets have more success in losing weight.

We will put legumes and beans in the same category, as most people think of them as the same thing, anyway. Beans are a notably good source of energy while somewhat paradoxically being low in calories. Much like potatoes, beans have been shown to be part of diets where people succeeded in losing weight.

You might already know this, but you still have to be somewhat careful with beans and legumes because they are high in carbs. But I still say they are good for intermittent fasting for all the reasons listed.

Now we are on to nuts. What makes this a great option is that they have unsaturated fats: the kind that you want. Specifically, nuts have polyunsaturated fats, just like olive oil. Walnut is one such example of a food with this healthy fat. You don't have to worry about the calories for nuts either, because for the healthy ones like walnuts, they usually end up being insignificant.

I don't want to spend too much time on vegetables because everyone knows that we are supposed to eat vegetables. But I will give you one more reason to eat them: they are packed with fiber. Of course, fiber aids in digestion, and autophagy aids in digestion too. When you combine your fiber from your vegetable-rich diet with intermittent fasting, your digestive system will be as healthy as it can be. Fiber is also great for intermittent fasting because it keeps you from feeling hungry during your fasting periods.

Avocados seem to be quite popular these days, but they really should be with IF practitioners. They are considered a "superfood" because they have a lot of the vitamins and nutrients that you need every day. Best of all, they have unsaturated fats. You can start eating a lot of avocados and get a lot of what you need from them so you can lower your caloric consumption.

While green tea may have chemicals that directly influence the power of autophagy, other teas could help with aspects of IF from a more pragmatic standpoint. For instance, while caffeine has been shown to help increase autophagy when it is triggered, if you get that caffeine from coffee, it will also help you feel fuller. Coffee or any kind of tea may have this effect on you.

Eat eggs, too. They have the protein that you need without a lot of the unhealthy stuff that tends to come with protein. And while we are talking about studies, there is research showing that people who replace a bagel with an egg feel less feelings of hunger during the day — so you might want to get into the habit of eating an egg every morning so you can have the best chances of succeeding with IF.

There you have it — the foods to eat and to leave out when you do IF. You can always check this chapter again if you're unsure what to do, but you should also learn to trust your instinct about what foods to eat.

You feel one way after eating a bag of Skittles and another after Brussels sprouts. You know which one is going to help you get these positive health effects from autophagy, and you know which one will hinder you.

Beware the tricks your mind will play on you to make you think that you are hungry for foods that do not even have essential nutrients. You can be sure this is just your brain trying to get the food you crave into your mouth.

Many people start the very first few hours into a fast and are convinced that they are already low on energy. True fatigue is one thing, but feeling a little tired after not eating for a couple of hours doesn't mean you need to eat a meal right away. You have to let feelings like this pass, or else they will seriously hinder your fast.

You are bound to feel like you are "slightly hungry" during your time doing the IF. This is something that you should expect with any fast after you spend your whole life never even contemplating it. Just be sure to know the difference between discomfort and pain — between unhealthy and "no pain, no gain."

Chapter 6:
Intermittent Fasting and Women

There is good reason to learn about intermittent fasting specifically as it applies to women because research has demonstrated that the IF has different effects on men and women. This is because women studied exhibited some less-than-desirable outcomes as a result of intermittent fasting. I tell you this to caution you about doing IF in a healthy way, not to scare you from doing something that would be good for your body.

Some women said their menstrual cycle altered because of IF, and some said their blood sugar went too low. Both of these outcomes can be avoided by consuming adequate nutrients when you are not fasting and by limiting your fasting times to reasonable windows.

All the success that women have been having with IF is the reason that it has gotten so popular suddenly. It's a pattern of eating that speaks to the health concerns that women are worried about: weight loss, risk of heart disease, risk of diabetes, and even risk of cancer.

While any person can do intermittent fasting, you know that women have their own specific issues that make their experience with IF different. But how exactly do their experiences differ?

It is just one study on laboratory mice, but there is one that showed that female mice who did concurrent day fasting for 3-6 had ovaries that were shrunk and irregular cycles, too.

One way is in the menstrual cycle and how it can interact with changes in diet. There has not been any scientific backing yet on if intermittent fasting can really affect your period, but there has definitely been a limited number of cases where women say their cycles were different, and they thought that IF was the cause.

It is hard to say if we can blame this entirely on the IF routine itself, though. Some have suggested that since women who do IF often want to lose weight, they are more likely to be overweight or obese. Being overweight

126

or obese is a risk factor for having irregular periods, so perhaps this is the cause of the irregular cycle during IF. However, we can't jump to conclusions.

But the menstrual cycle is not the only thing that women have to consider when doing IF that men don't. Their hormones are also different and affecting their eating habits differently.

These hormone differences give some credence to the idea that intermittent fasting can have negative consequences for women if you are not careful. The main hormone in the spotlight is GnRH, which is affected when women consume fewer calories.

If women consume too few calories, their GnRH might be interrupted, which could put them at risk for irregular periods.

We do have to keep in mind that this is a side effect of low caloric intake, not intermittent fasting. Women who want to lose weight, to some extent, do just have to consume fewer calories. These women may accept the temporary changes to their period, knowing that their weight loss will have many positive, long-lasting benefits.

There may still be something to the idea that women should think about their specific issues when choosing to do intermittent fasting. They might choose to fast for a shorter period of time and for fewer days.

If we are being honest, while anyone can do an intermittent fast to get the health benefits of autophagy, most of the people who are doing it are women. The science showing women some of the woman-specific problems that come with IF shouldn't scare them from doing it. They should keep doing it anyway because the initial discomfort is worth the payoff they will get when they lose weight, have better skin, and have a detoxified system.

Doctors know that women have reproductive systems that are closely related to their metabolisms. This makes sense because when women are carrying children, they have to be able to feed them from the inside.

Even if you aren't pregnant, however, the deep entanglement between the female reproductive system and the female metabolism affects your body. When you have not had a period for a while during the same time that you changed your pattern of eating, there is a greater-than-luck chance that your missing period is because of your fasting.

You don't want to give up on IF just because it can be hard as a woman. You need to take the challenge and do the thing that is good for your body, even when it puts you through some periods of discomfort.

Remember that hormone changes are fleeting, so if you experience a change in hormones during the time that you fast, it doesn't mean that the fast is bad for you. Over time, they will adjust until it is just another part of your day.

Getting used to it will be a matter of managing your stress and sleep. Mostly, you want to pay attention to your stress, but your stress is connected to a whole list of things. They include not eating enough calories, not getting enough nutrients, not being active enough, chronic inflammation, and finally, sleep deprivation.

If you can manage all of these things, your hormones should not give you too much of a trouble as you transition into IF.

Nonetheless, going for an extended period of time without a period could be a sign of something serious. If this happens, you should stop your fast and schedule a doctor's visit.

Intermittent Fasting and Women: Made for Each Other

Don't let the anecdotal stories about irregular cycles make you afraid of doing what will ultimately be good for you. If you are being honest with yourself, at least part of the reason you would think IF could be harmful to women is so you don't have to do the work to get autophagy's benefits.

In all truth, autophagy is a wonderful way that women can take control of their bodies. Every woman on Earth wants a sustainable way to lose weight, increase muscle mass, and rev up their energy. The autophagy women get from triggering autophagy with intermittent fasting comes with all of these rewards, so it's no wonder so many women are talking about IF.

As you know well, autophagy also confers long-term health benefits, but some of them are particularly important to women: a more acute stress response from their cells so that autophagy is easier to trigger in the future, improved sensitivity to insulin, and an increase in the growth hormone, which is vital to many processes that your body goes through.

With all of these positives from intermittent fasting, it wouldn't be wise to completely ignore some of the indications that IF can interfere with the female reproductive system, too. But that only means we need to be measured in the way we trigger autophagy. It doesn't mean we abandon IF altogether.

I am not saying that women should never do a full, 24-hour extended water fast. However, if you ever experience any signs that IF influences your cycle, then it might be a good idea to avoid that long of a fast. It might be better for you to fast for around 12 hours instead.

Since you don't yet know how your body will react to fasting as a woman until you have done it, I also advise you to start very slow with your first fast. You probably should not even fast for two days in a row during your first week, if you really want to be careful.

There are some groups of women that should not do intermittent fasting altogether. If you have had a history of problems with any major organs, such as your lungs, heart, or liver, you should not do intermittent fasting. It could put too much stress on these organs, and the potential benefit you would get from IF would not be enough to justify you harming them.

It should be obvious that pregnant women should not fast. As I have said, the female reproductive system is closely tied to the woman's metabolism. When that woman is with child, she doesn't have the luxury of purposefully depriving herself of nutrients to trigger autophagy anymore, because now the health of her body and of her child is what determines her health the most.

Sadly, there are many women with eating disorders compared to men. Women who have or who have had eating disorders should not attempt to do intermittent fasting. They are at too high a risk of losing any progress they might have made in establishing normal eating patterns.

My final two tips for women who do IF are the same ones I have said throughout our book: drink a lot of water and exercise. Both of these activities will keep your body in shape so it can handle the stress of autophagy and IF better.

Chapter 7:

Intermittent Fasting for Women over 50

Overweight women over 50 have a higher risk of diabetes and heart problems than they did when they were younger. IF is one option they have to manage their weight and control these health risks.

The metabolism of a woman over 50 has become slower, so you can't expect quick results if you are a member of this group, but you will probably get the most out of it than any other group of women because of all the anti-aging effects of IF and autophagy.

Overweight and obese people have higher risks of heart disease, stroke, and more as they age. On the other hand, thinner people are not looking at these same risks.

Losing weight can only be good for your body, and autophagy is the healthiest and most effective way to do it. Autophagy will help you stay thin, feel good, and be healthy for years and years.

But, so far, we have only talked about the health benefits that are immediately obvious. There is also a reduction of health risks that are not cosmetic like youthful skin and weight loss. It has been proven that an increase in autophagy reduces your risk of Alzheimer's and Parkinson's disease.

More autophagy also reduces inflammation, which will increase your overall health. There has even been research about the benefits of autophagy for cancer patients undergoing chemotherapy.

Studies have shown that cancer patients going through chemotherapy saw a reduction in the clumps of white blood cells that accumulate because of chemotherapy. Dead cells can be hazardous to your body if they are not cleaned out during autophagy.

Since these patients fasted in order to turn on autophagy, their bodies were able to clean out the white blood cells and recover from chemotherapy sooner.

You can only imagine the kind of advantage you get if you are turning autophagy on as much as possible, and you aren't even looking at a major health risk yet. You may not have as big an accumulation of dead cells as someone going through chemotherapy, but if you have not fasted before and you don't exercise regularly, it is very likely that you have a lot of toxins in your body.

This is because if you don't go through autophagy very often, materials like dead cells, dead organelles, and unused proteins start to pile up and make your cells less efficient.

Putting your body through autophagy doesn't just combat aging in ways that are immediately visible. It also greatly reduces your risk of long-term age-related disease. Whether you're looking to improve the quality of your life or the length of your life, making autophagy happen in your body will do it.

There are many misconceptions about how autophagy does its anti-aging work. Perhaps the most common is that its only health benefits come from taking care of toxins. Clearing toxins from your system is certainly a good thing, but autophagy goes far beyond ridding your body of harmful chemicals.

Most of these toxins are not from outside your body, but they are materials like proteins and organelles that your cells used once and then no longer had a use for. These discarded materials start to take up space over time, creating clutter that slows down your cells. This is when they become toxins.

Some of these toxins cause even worse problems than congestion. The worst case is protein clusters that form in the brain. Neurodegenerative diseases like Alzheimer's become more of a concern as we age, and autophagy might be your best ally in fighting against your risk of these diseases.

From a broader perspective, Alzheimer's manifests as "knots" and "tangles" in the brain that impair memory.

When doctors look at the knots and tangles with a microscope, they see that these irregularities are actually clusters of proteins that have built up over time. They are proteins that brain cells used at one point but later had no purpose. The protein clusters were not managed with autophagy, so they simply accumulated and started leading to serious memory problems.

Alzheimer's disease is the most extreme consequence that you can have from not going through enough autophagy. It is not the only consequence, however. Discarded materials like protein clusters start to build up throughout your body if you rarely go through autophagy.

In this regard, low autophagy leads to a low count of collagen, the protein that makes your skin youthful. Your skin cells can't produce collagen when they are crowded by cellular garbage.

Similarly, you lose more muscle mass if you rarely go through autophagy because you are not turning on autophagy to repair the muscle tissue damage that results from physical activity.

From these examples alone, you can see that autophagy is more than a toxin-cleaning agent. Autophagy doesn't only destroy the bad (toxins); it builds the good (new organelles, proteins, and cells). Both sides of autophagy make it such a powerful anti-aging tool, one that was surprisingly given to us by nature.

So far, we have established that autophagy isn't just good for destroying pathogen invaders — it also destroys materials that become toxic when they linger in the cell for too long. In short, this biological process cleans out toxins from the outside and inside.

In the third stage, your cells use these broken-down parts as ingredients to build new cells and cell structures. What's more: your cells have more room to build new cells and new cell parts because they freed up so much space during autophagy.

All these things come together when you find a way to turn on autophagy on a regular basis. Equipped with all this information, you know much more about autophagy than even your average fasting practitioner.

Women over 50 certainly still want to manage their weight and have good skin, but it is around this age that we start to get a more mature perspective on life, and we care more about the health consequences of our daily life choices than before. They have many options for unlocking autophagy even further than they would with IF alone.

Back in the 90s, the idea of caloric restriction became very popular, and people saw improvements in their health from doing nothing more than eating less. There is even a great deal of evidence that mammals who restrict their calories live longer than mammals who do not.

This has not yet been proven to be true for humans, but still, restricting your caloric intake can only be a good thing. You get this additional benefit from turning on autophagy through fasting while also getting the benefit of autophagy itself along with it.

We have heard a lot of ideas about losing weight from nutritionists in the last few decades, but let's not kid ourselves: the main reason for weight gain across the planet comes down to people consuming a lot of calories without physically exerting themselves to burn them off. Fasting for any length of time will lead to consuming fewer calories, so you are on the right track for losing weight when you fast.

The next popular method of turning on autophagy is the keto diet. This method will turn on autophagy because it involves depriving your body of nutrients that it would normally consume for energy.

However, following the keto diet alone will not turn on autophagy because it is only activated when your cells are in a state of stress, and as long as you are sedentary or filling your body with any kind of food, your cells are not in this state.

That said, since the keto diet is so low in carbs, this style of eating will aid in turning on autophagy. I definitely recommend following the keto diet because the mistake many autophagy practitioners make is consuming a lot of carbs while they are not fasting.

Eating a lot of carbs will prevent your body from fasting for a long time because it takes a long time for your digestive system to process them. Not only that, but as you may be aware, it becomes harder to keep weight off the older you get, and you are significantly slowing down the process of burning fat when your digestive tract has a backlog of carbs. Fighting against this problem is the role of the keto diet in anti-aging and autophagy.

Next, there is the method of good old exercise. Studies have shown that resistance training, also known as strength training, is the most effective way of turning on autophagy, saying it is even more effective than fasting. The reason for this is that when you use your muscles, you are getting tiny tears in your muscle tissue that are repaired through autophagy.

The unfortunate thing is that exercising might be the last thing that people want to do, even though it is so good for their health. Like the other methods, exercise has its own health benefits that are separate from autophagy.

Plenty of studies show that people who work out regularly have lower risks of all age-related illnesses, even those not related to the heart. If we are being honest, exercising is probably the best way to fight aging.

If you want to get the most out of autophagy, you should employ all of these methods together. When combined, the keto diet, exercise, and fasting will give you the greatest benefits, both in terms of weight loss and in general health.

If you don't yet feel motivated to be as healthy as possible, try to think of the autophagy in your cells as an analogy for your personal health. If they did not recycle their cellular garbage, your cells would simply die after their organelles stopped working or they were overcrowded with protein clusters and foreign invaders.

If you do not recycle your body's toxins by turning on autophagy regularly, your body will be over-encumbered with cellular garbage and you will be less healthy as a result. If this analogy were expanded, you might even live a shorter life if you do not regularly clean out your cellular garbage via autophagy.

Your cells try to live longer by using autophagy to combat their cellular aging — you should try to use autophagy to work against aging too.

Chapter 8:
Intermittent Fasting
Techniques: 16/8, Keto Diet,
and More

After talking a little bit about the different ways that women do intermittent fasting, and now it's time to go into them in detail. The first one, and maybe the most well-known, is 16/8 intermittent fasting.

The fundamental aspect of IF — not eating for some period of the day — is easily observed in 16/8. You only eat for 8 hours of the day, and you fast for the other 16 hours. It is also typical for IF practitioners to follow the keto diet, a low-carb diet designed to induce ketosis in your body to help in burning body fat.

Many women get confused about what intermittent fasting requires of them because they are used to following diets, not fasts. IF is a new pattern of eating, not a diet. There are foods that you should eat in an IF fast since they help with the goal of autophagy, as we learned in Chapter 5. But IF itself is no diet.

The other side of that is women thinking they can eat anything since it is not a diet. This is obviously not true either

In one sense, intermittent fasting is simpler than dieting. You could say it's simpler because you are not basing all of your health and body goals on eating certain foods and restricting others. On a fundamental level, the most important thing to do for the IF is to commit to not eating for a number of hours at the same time every day.

But you could also say that it is more complicated, because its advocates — me included — will not make the claim that fasting alone will do everything. The truth is, the IF itself is doing most of the work, but you will only see the results if you adopt habits that are good for your health, too.

That said, I hope this book has given you a good sense of how autophagy ties into all aspects of health, because it really does tie into intermittent fasting, working out, and eating healthy.

The point we are trying to come to is that you could work out every day and eat all of the foods you are supposed to eat, but not fast; you would be healthy, without a doubt. But on balance, you probably wouldn't be as healthy as someone who worked out a little less, ate a little less healthy, but did intermittent fasting every day.

That's because autophagy is the vital cellular process your whole body relies upon, but that people do not pay nearly enough attention to.

You are nearing the end of the book, and that means it's time to put together your plan of attack for this fast. What kind are you going to do? Whichever one you choose, you should write down your exact goal for the number of hours you want to fast and the date you will start.

When the day comes, mark the actual time you start fasting and the actual time you stop. Write down whether you "cheat" during your fasting window or not. Keeping a log like this will make it a lot more likely for you to do IF successfully.

The 12-Hour Fast

This intermittent fast is a good one to start with, although if the idea of fasting is completely new to you and makes you nervous, you are totally free to reduce it to 10 hours or less.

The trick for a simple intermittent fast like this is to ensure you are still getting the healthy number of calories every day but to simply get them outside of the 12-hour long window that you have decided to fast for.

The 12-hour fast is also a good place to start for someone who wants to end up doing a more ambitious fast. You don't start so low that going as high as 16 hours seems infeasible. You may even want to work up to a 20-hour fast if you are feeling bold, though, at that point, you may want to consider trying the 24-hour water fast.

The times during which you fast are entirely up to you. Any intermittent fast is best done by waking up relatively early, eating breakfast, fasting, and then eating dinner not too soon before bed. You don't want to eat too close to your bedtime because then you will be spending a lot of your precious autophagy time during sleep by breaking down your food.

It is surprising that we have not even had the opportunity to talk about the importance of sleep with autophagy.

There are some facts about sleep and autophagy that you need to seriously consider.

You do the most autophagy that you do throughout your day when you are sleeping. Even in people who do not think about fasting or autophagy whatsoever, their highest level of autophagy is when they are sleeping, and so is yours.

That means when you eat really close to the time you go to bed — let's say you eat at 7pm and then sleep at 9pm — you aren't giving your body enough time to break down your food. You don't have any significant autophagy when you are digesting, so digesting in your sleep is a big wasted opportunity.

Even the 12-hour fast can prove challenging, because you don't want to wake up too unreasonably early, but you don't want to digest food during the time that you should be going through advanced autophagy while you are asleep, either.

You may choose to wake up and eat your first meal at 7am. 12 hours later, your fast is over, and you eat dinner at 7pm. You can probably already see how this can problematic; if you get enough sleep to wake up at 7am, you will want to be in bed by 10pm. However, this does leave 3 hours between your dinner and your bedtime, so while it is a tight squeeze, this system does work out for the 12-hour fast.

The 8-Hour Fast

You could call this a beginner fast. That doesn't mean that it's a small feat, though. Don't forget that IF is every day. 8 hours may not seem like a long time to go without food, but if you haven't done it before, doing it every day might end up being a lot harder than you expected.

Some call the 16-hour fast the "16:8 diet," so you can call this one the "8:16 diet," if you like. As you can see, leaving plenty of time between dinner and sleep is a lot easier with this diet. You can eat dinner at 6pm, go to bed at 10pm, wake up at 7am, and get your nutrients between then and 10am. But between 10am and 6pm, you are doing your intermittent fast.

It is funny how compared to the 12-hour fast the 8-hour fast seems like it is a small feat, but when you get down to what is expected, it is still a hard thing for many people to do — especially every day.

The 5:2 Fast

Not every kind of intermittent fasting is based around the number of hours you fast every day. In earnest, I recommend doing the traditional 8-hour fast to start out and simply make it longer as you become more comfortable. However, I have said throughout the book that you have the freedom to do whatever works for you and your body — so it would be a disservice to you if I didn't let you know what other options are out there for IF.

In 5:2, you eat the way you would normally for five days of the week (still eating healthy, though). During the other two days, women only consume 500 calories.

The usual guidance applies — you don't get to glut out on your non-fasting days just because you aren't in a fast. You will want to make sure you get all the nutrients you need on the non-fasting days, though, because you won't be able to cram many important ones into 500 calories on those days.

There are some people who think 5:2 would work better for them because they can't imagine committing to fasting every single day of the week. With 5:2, you do an extreme fast for two days of the week so that you don't have to fast at all on most days of the week.

Concurrent Day Fasting

This kind of fast itself has different versions to it, but they all follow the basic idea of fasting every other day instead of every single day. It is similar to the 5:2 fast, except you don't have to go as extreme on your fasting days.

Concurrent day fasting, sometimes called alternate day fasting, has been tested in some studies, and people did have luck in losing weight when following it. The main drawback of it is that people say they never feel entirely full when following it.

If you want to follow concurrent day fasting yourself, you don't have to do much to plan it out. Of course, you eat on whatever schedule you normally would on your non-fasting days, and then every other day you fast.

Since you aren't fasting every day, you need to consider that when deciding how long you will go. You don't want to do an 8-hour fast, because that is too short, considering that you will go back to not fasting the next day. A 12- or 16-hour fast might work, depending on your experience with fasting so far.

You have no shortage of options for intermittent fasting. I hope you feel that thanks to this book, you are at no shortage of information, either.

You may feel somewhat overwhelmed after reading guide to intermittent fasting that is so chockfull of information. The Table of Contents may be helpful to you in case you think you should revisit a topic again.

Conclusion

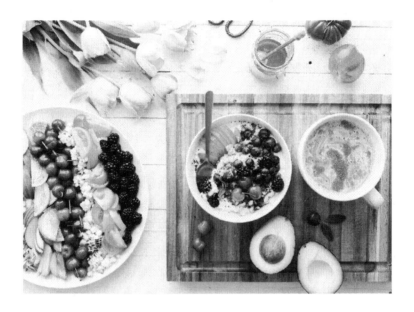

Thank you for making it through to the end of *Intermittent Fasting for Women 101*, let's hope it was informative and able to provide you with all of the tools you need to achieve your goals whatever they may be.

After being exposed to so much knowledge about intermittent fasting, you aren't likely to be surprised by the fact that the American Heart Association recommends intermittent fasting for losing weight. Its effectiveness in helping women lose weight is backed by science as well as by the personal experiences of thousands of women.

Fasting has existed in religious traditions for millennia, and now anyone can harness its health benefits with intermittent fasting. You don't have to undergo nearly the level of physical and mental fatigue of traditional water fasts, but you still see the difference in your waistline and in how you feel.

The scientific credibility that intermittent fasting has is all thanks to the biological process of autophagy. Autophagy is your body's natural means of getting rid of toxins that pollute your system. Intermittent fasting is your means of triggering this vital process.

Biologists have been studying autophagy and its revelatory implications for health heavily in the last ten years — and some of the most important findings have been in just the last few years! Be sure to check out the appendix at the end of the book so you can learn more about what scientists are finding out.

The more and more mainstream attention that autophagy has been receiving can be attributed to the research of Nobel Prize-winning Yoshinori Ohsumi. He is the scientist who studied autophagy in yeast cells for decades and was finally recognized for his important work.

His research led to more scientists studying the role of autophagy in fighting cancer and age-related disease. What has been found is that triggering autophagy on purpose can help us live healthier lives, longer lives, and more youthful lives.

Intermittent fasting is your ticket into triggering autophagy because it is easy to sustain. Unlike other means of achieving autophagy, intermittent fasting doesn't ask that you go to the gym or change what you eat (although you should still these things to get the most out of the biological process). Start your intermittent fast today and you will see all the health benefits uncovered in this book for yourself.

If you're still skeptical, make sure to peruse the appendix, which is filled with scientific studies on intermittent fasting done by experts.

Finally, if you found this book useful in any way, a review on Amazon is always appreciated!

From the same Author

Intermittent Fasting Diet Guide: *A Complete Step-By-Step Guide for Heal Your Body, Weight Loss, Fat Burn and Live in a Healthy and Happy Way with the Autophagy Process **(Meal Plan with 60 Recipes).***

Cook, J. (2019 Nov 17).

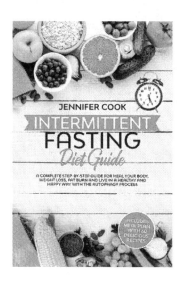

Autophagy: *For Women and Men who Desire to Purify their Body, Lose Weight, and Slow Aging with a Natural Self-Cleaning Metabolic Process using Extended Water, Intermittent Fasting and a Ketogenic Diet.*

Cook, J. (2020 Dec 03).

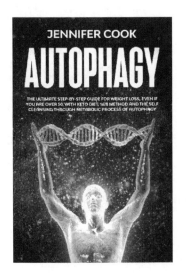

Appendix: Studies on Intermittent Fasting and Autophagy

Anton, Moehl, Donahoo, Marosi, Lee, et al. *Flipping the Metabolic Switch: Understanding and Applying Health Benefits of Fasting*. 2017 Oct 31. ncbi.nlm.nih.gov/pmc/articles/PMC5783752/

This study focuses on the physical effects of intermittent fasting on the most important organs of the body. The authors conclude that lowering the level of glucose in your body can actually aid in keeping your muscle mass. They say this can be a boon for people who are struggling with their weight. They even conclude that fasting results in the activation of neural pathways with a lot of great effects, in including fighting aging and slow the progression of disease.

Bartosz, Zalewska, Wesierska, Sokolowska, et al. *Intermittent Fasting in Cardiovascular Disorders—An Overview.* Published 2019 Mar 20. ncbi.nlm.nih.gov/pmc/articles/PMC6471315/

The authors conclude that doing intermittent fasting greatly reduces the risk of getting a cardiovascular disease. Participants in this eating pattern are able to maintain a source of energy through fatty acids and ketones while the body goes through metabolic switching between glucose and ketones. These scientists even conclude that intermittent fasting helps people lose body mass by changing the transformations of your lipids. They also say that it reduces cholesterol in its practitioners.

Antunes, Erustes, Costa, Nascimento, et al. *Autophagy and intermittent fasting: the connection for cancer therapy?* Published 2018 Nov 27. ncbi.nlm.nih.gov/pmc/articles/PMC6257056/

These authors examine the role that autophagy can play in fighting against cancer. They write that autophagy can either help cancer cells grow or help non-cancerous cells grow to fight against them, depending on the situation.

They consider the possible use of autophagy for fighting tumors. Fasting in particular is outlined as the chief strategy in using autophagy to fight cancer. The main conclusion is the use of autophagy for protecting non-cancerous cells from toxic cancer cells as well as for reducing the side effects from chemotherapy.

Ganesan, Habboush, Sultan. *Intermittent Fasting: The Choice for a Healthier Lifestyle.* Published online 2018 Jul 9. ncbi.nlm.nih.gov/pmc/articles/PMC6128599/

A meta-analysis of studies done in the past 20 years on the subject of intermittent fasting. Not only did these studies show that people who did intermittent fasting lost weight, but they also improved on important biological measures like reduced low-density lipoprotein and triglyceride. No matter the body type of the studies' participants, they succeeded in losing weight on average.

Harvie, Howell. *Potential Benefits and harms of Intermittent Energy Restriction and Intermittent Fasting Amongst Obese, Overweight and Normal Weight Subjects—A Narrative Review of Human and Animal*

Evidence. Published 2017 Jan 19. ncbi.nlm.nih.gov/pmc/articles/PMC5371748/

These authors go over and compare experiments on intermittent fasting and intermittent energy restriction (referred to in this book as caloric restriction). Their findings are that there is no real evidence of either method being harmful, and while both methods show promise for helping people lose weight, fasting is more consistently effective. They note that there is a lack of research on the effective of intermittent fasting and caloric restriction on people who are not overweight or obese.

Jacomin, Gul, Sudhakar, Korcsmaros, Nezis. *What We Learned from Big Data for Autophagy Research.* Published 2018 Aug 17. ncbi.nlm.nih.gov/pmc/articles/PMC6107789/

The scientists went into this study wanting to investigate the relation between autophagy and other integral cellular processes. They use big data to do an overview of what biologists have learned about this relation. The authors find that autophagy plays an important part in many different pathologies, including in infections and in cancer. Its role in neurodegenerative diseases is also well-known.

Yoshii, Mizushima. *Monitoring and Measuring Autophagy*. 2017 Sep 18. ncbi.nlm.nih.gov/pmc/articles/PMC5618514/

Yoshii and Mizushima examine a number of meta issues in studying autophagy, including the use of mice and their anatomical closeness to humans and the accuracy of the results in studies that use samples to make conclusions about autophagy in human beings.

Made in the USA
Middletown, DE
20 February 2020

85080955R00091